How We See Ourselves

This light-hearted and entertaining book, authored by top psychologist David Cohen, explores the influences and impacts on our perception of body image, examining the power of appearance and the psychology behind how we think and feel about ourselves physically.

Packed with scientific findings alongside historical anecdotes and humorous insights, the book first looks at the history of body image and appearance, and how ideals of beauty have changed over time. It goes on to note the rise of the beauty and fashion industries, looking at how society, culture and the media can affect body image. The final section deals with issues of body dissatisfaction and the treatments and therapy available for those struggling with body image and mental health. Along the way, readers will meet a cast of characters from Elizabeth I, a daring, medieval Welsh poet, an Egyptian mummy with the first known tattoo, Paul F. Schilder who pioneered the study of body image, and the brave recipients of the first face transplants, among many more.

In his trademark engaging style, Cohen offers a rich account of the psychology of body image through the ages and through the lifespan. It is valuable reading for students of psychology and professionals and therapists aiming to promote body positivity.

David Cohen is a psychologist, film maker, and a Fellow of the Royal Society of Medicine. His film about the Soham murders, When Holly Went Missing, was nominated for a BAFTA award.

How We See Ourselves

How Psychology, Society and the Media Affect Our Body Image

David Cohen

Routledge
Taylor & Francis Group
LONDON AND NEW YORK

First published 2025
by Routledge
4 Park Square, Milton Park, Abingdon, Oxon OX14 4RN

and by Routledge
605 Third Avenue, New York, NY 10158

Routledge is an imprint of the Taylor & Francis Group, an informa business

Designed cover image: Getty images via microgen

British Library Cataloguing in Publication Data
A catalogue record for this book is available from the British Library

Library of Congress Cataloging-in-Publication Data
A catalog record has been requested for this book

ISBN: 978-1-032-54632-2 (hbk)
ISBN: 978-1-032-54628-5 (pbk)
ISBN: 978-1-003-42587-8 (ebk)

DOI: 10.4324/9781003425878

Typeset in
by Taylor & Francis Books

Contents

Contents

Introduction

Mirror, mirror on the wall – who's the fairest of them all?

Narcissus did not need a mirror to adore himself. He just looked in the nearby pond. Thinking himself utterly beautiful he never said, 'I must improve my looks.' He seems like vanity personified but Benjamin Franklin, one of the founding fathers of America, seems to have had a soft spot for him, as we shall see.

Authors often list the demographics their book should interest. This one should be useful to psychologists and psychiatrists, as well as to those interested in fashion but, reader, do you have a body? If so, this book is for you.

This is not a self-help book, but readers may find it helpful to stand in front of a mirror, strip, and look at their body. Carefully. Work out what you like or dislike about what you see. Brave readers may ask their partners, if they have one, what they like or dislike about their body. Remember bodies change and those changes may affect feelings. The meta-verse, which sometimes feels like the meta-worse these days, also is relevant. Do you have an avatar? Do you plan to leave a digital twin to console your loved one when you pop your binaries and go to the great i.cloud?

Very few of us are totally satisfied with our bodies. So, we adorn them to make them look more powerful, more attractive, even more intellectual. Sex shops offer many tantalising devices. Perhaps the most dramatic is the penis enlarger, which does not come just in flesh colours, but also in sexy pink with stripes. Lovehoney is the name of one such brand.

But there are less salacious ways to change the way you look, like:

Mascara
False eyelashes

Nail polish
Nail extensions (including the Dracula 500 Pieces Medium Long Stiletto Straight Pointed False Nail Tips NATURAL Full Cover Acrylic Press On False Nails Tips Extensions)
Rings in your nose, ears, lips, and navel. (Some people put rings in their genitals, which sounds painful.)
There must be research on rings in enlarged penises but that is perhaps not vital to cover this.

Let us now praise capitalism and the Beauty Industry, which trills that you are never too young to use make-up. Amazon offers their 5 PCS REAL KIDS MAKE-UP SET INCLUDES: 1x Makeup case with mirror, 12x Matte Eyeshadow, 8x Glitter Eyeshadows, 4x Sequin Eyeshadow, 4x Nail Polish, 3x Lipsticks, 1x Powder, 4x Blush, 1x Cosmetic Sponge, 1x Toe Separator, 1x Nail File, 11x Makeup Brush.

"This is a makeup set girl toys designed for girls, small and delicate. Each of the makeup accessories has a separate location so Mom does not have to worry about messy. The hand case is very useful when, after putting on make-up, they want to put everything back in place, or even to take make-up on the road."

This might make little children happy, but should they really be using make-up so young?

Don't forget the philosophy. Amazon trills "Loving beauty is the nature of everyone, and children are no exception. Our washable Girls makeup toys can satisfy children's curiosity and beauty, and at the same time, it can cultivate and improve children's creativity, imagination and learning ability while enjoying the fun."

Let's continue the list.

Glasses and sunglasses. Sunglasses often seem glamorous. but ordinary glasses are supposed to be off-putting. 'Men don't make passes at girls who wear glasses', it has been said by the American poet, Dorothy Parker, but there are now dozens of stylish glasses which sparkle allure. In the wonderful film *How to Marry a Millionaire* Marilyn Monroe plays a blind-as-a-bat blonde, who tries not to wear glasses, as she thinks that will make her look unattractive. In my opinion, to make Marilyn look unattractive you would have to paint a Cubist image of her. So, it appears that glasses can make someone look dull, bookish, or stunning.

We use the following beauty top-ups too:

Haircuts of every sort

Hair extensions

Waxes, which leave what some women call a landing strip. Tattoos range from a tiny bird on your ankle to what I shall call the Full

Monty, where almost the whole body is covered. Body painting may have been the earliest form of art – ochre was being used at least 200,000 years ago in Africa and Europe, and Neanderthals were daubing themselves with pigment to look flash as long as 60,000 years ago. And maybe dancing at the same time.

Body image is a sprawling subject covering alopecia to zombies. It involves questions of our sense of identity, such as face transplants or body dysmorphia, which can lead to mental health problems. As a result, this book covers many issues. But body image can also be funny, as it shows how vain humans can be – and how they can upset their dearest and nearest if they look scruffy. P.G. Wodehouse created Lord Emsworth, the elderly absent-minded owner of Blandings Castle. They might not let Lord Emsworth into the House of Lords as he looks more like a tramp than a peer, but his life is full of unwanted drama. He has to rescue his dim-witted son Freddie, thwart pig thieves, and enable young lovers to marry. His sisters, however, think he looks a mess, which annoys him, as he just wants to be left in peace to devote himself to his prize pig, Empress of Blandings, who is his true love and will never be turned into a pork chop while he is alive.

I admire Woodhouse, so in his spirit, this book also introduces the fictional rabbi's wife who was always nagging him to wash properly, wash the dishes, and comb the lice out of his beard.

Most body image research has been carried out on students, but there has been some research on the body image of certain groups including disabled athletes, gymnasts, and dancers, who have particular body image attitudes. I quote personal accounts a few times, because they often reveal how difficult it is when you are not at ease with your body image.

Poets have praised beautiful women since the Greeks. I thought first that I would have a whole chapter on those. Instead, I have put poetry at relevant points throughout including a rude Welsh woman poet who marvelled at her genitals in brilliant verse.

As the book deals with a variety of themes it may help readers to have an outline of the chapters:

- Chapter 1 sets the scene by discussing the four basic components of body image. I dare to add a fifth – our unconscious body image.
- Chapter 2 looks at body image ideals through the ages from the ancient Greeks to the beauty salons of the 1930s, via a brief history of corsets. It also looks at the golden ratio, the proportions on the face and body which are seen as utterly beautiful, as discussed by Leonardo da Vinci.

- Chapter 3 looks at the academic study of body image, beginning with the work of Paul Schilder, the psychoanalyst who pioneered the study of body image– and tangled with Freud. It also looks at the work of the French psychoanalyst Francoise Dolto and discusses the many tests of body image.
- Chapter 4 examines the influence of social media on body image.
- Chapter 5 continues this theme, through an exploration of the effects of other media and celebrities on body image, particularly among adolescents. It examines the research on how teenagers see themselves and react to criticism of their looks.
- Chapter 6 looks at case histories of eating disorders, body image disturbance and body dysmorphia and what can help – and how effectively.
- Chapter 7 examines fitness, dieting, and the wellness business.
- Chapter 8 looks at how we have adorned our bodies with tattoos and body piercing.
- Chapter 9 explores facial disfigurement and one of the most radical changes in body image – face transplants.
- Chapter 10 looks at disability and body image.
- This book started out as a book on hair. Chapter 11 looks at the significance of hair, and unwanted hair, on body image. It includes a history of beards and the regulations for the unlikely world moustache competition.
- Chapter 12 examines baldness – its causes and consequences – and takes a closer look at alopecia and other hair trauma, such as sudden changes of colour.
- Chapter 13 examines body image as we age. We are living longer, and in 2024 there were some 500,000 90-year-olds in the UK. How we view ourselves as we get older is often a list of painful changes.
- Finally, I offer a personal appendix.

Personal

As this book is not just academic but personal, I confess that I have hair and body image problems. When I was 13, I was not just podgy, but I thought that all my hair was falling out. I saved money and went to see a hair doctor – the official designation is a trichologist, a specialist in the treatment of the hair and scalp.

The trichologist sighed and said that I was one of the worst cases he'd ever seen. If I didn't buy his super ointment, I'd be bald before I was 20. No girl would look at me. Ever. I bought the ointment, of course, and applied it, of course. For months.

Sixty years on I'm proud of my hair. I have had less success with flab though.

My mother Dolly grew up in the 1920s, when physical culture was popular in Europe. She kept on telling me to slim, so that I would be rid of my *Bauch* – German for stomach. She did gymnastic exercises every day and nagged me to follow her example. She had never hoped to be a ballet dancer or a gymnast but did some 30 minutes of exercises every day. My father made fun of her obsession with physical fitness and of her use of laxatives. I watched her with admiration when I was a boy, but I had not the slightest intention of imitating her routines.

She loved the phrase *mens sano in corpore sano* (a healthy body in a healthy mind). I grew up imagining that the Romans muttered this every day as they wallowed in their baths while slaves scrubbed their backs and read the latest Cicero to them.

She didn't give up on me though. When I was older, she often nagged me to swim, run, play tennis, go to the gym. A paper on going to the gym and sadism is needed.

"Later," I always used to say, "when I've got time."

I never had time. Once I left school, I did no sports. The only time I did any strenuous exercise was the morning after I had gone to see a ballet based on Ravel's *Bolero*. The lead dancer swung and swivelled as Ravel's beat got faster and faster. The next day by some coincidence *Bolero* was on the radio. I got up and started gyrating as the astonishing dancer whose name I still remember – Jorge Lavelli – had done the night before.

I knew that I was no dancer, but I felt exhilarated as I did it. Bodies can give us joy – something to remember as we consider body image.

Then there is the Agatha Christie problem. The plot of one of her books *Dumb Witness* turns on the fact that Poirot realises – his little grey cells must have been having a nap – that what you see in a mirror is a reversed image, so when a witness sees a woman in a dressing gown on which A.T is embroidered, the dressing gown belongs to someone whose initials are really T.A., who is the killer, of course. "Mirror, mirror on the wall" may sound good, but you don't really see your body in the mirror. People tend to be anxious about their looks, but they don't really see themselves accurately. Psychology has tended to ignore this snag.

1 The Components of Body Image

Psychologists dissect body image into four components: perceptual, affective, cognitive and behavioural. Your perceptions, beliefs, feelings, thoughts, and actions make up your body image which is your personal relationship with your personal body. This implies that you have a lot of control over your body image but that is not always the case.

1. Perceptual

According to the National Eating Disorders Collaboration, "The way you see your body is your perceptual body image. This is not always a correct representation of how you actually look." Someone may see themselves as overweight when they are extremely thin – and that distortion can lead to eating disorders.

Our sometimes warped self-perception affects our well-being, as a 2021 Mental Health Foundation survey found. A total of 34 per cent of adults said they felt anxious or depressed because of their body image; just over one in eight experienced suicidal thoughts or feelings because of concerns about how they looked. A second survey of 1,118 British teenagers found that 40 per cent felt worried, 37 per cent felt upset, and 31 per cent felt ashamed in relation to their body image.

Those who suffer from 'higher body dissatisfaction' tend to be more depressed, to have a poorer quality of life, to eat unhealthily and have more eating disorders. It's a vicious circle. You feel low, you grab some chocolate or some celery if you are trying to eat healthy. Few of us have never succumbed to comfort eating.

DOI: 10.4324/9781003425878-1

Alice ten feet tall

Writing a book is an adventure and in writing this I have stumbled on one of the greatest – Alice in Wonderland. Lewis Carroll's story has led to a neurological condition – the Alice in Wonderland syndrome:

Anne Weissenstein, Elisabeth Luchter, and Stefan Bittmann take us down the rabbit hole (2015). This is a syndrome where your perception changes so that the sizes of body parts or sizes of external objects are perceived incorrectly. The most common perceptions are at night.

The authors saw a six-year-old boy who showed no brain abnormalities but still often experienced false perceptions lasting 15 to 20 minutes.

More often than not, the head and hands seem disproportionate, and usually, the person perceives growth of various parts rather than a reduction in their size. The patient often perceives the sizes of various other objects inaccurately and also loses a sense of time. Time seems passing either at a snail's pace or too swiftly. Some people experience strong hallucinations.

Temporal lobe epilepsy is another causal factor. The authors suggest that 15 per cent of children get the condition. The individual may get terrified, anxious and panic-stricken. The good news is that in all likelihood the distortions will fade over a period of time.

2. Affective

The way you feel about your body, especially how satisfied or dissatisfied you are about your looks, is your affective body image. Introducing a new edition of *Body Image*, Grogan (2021) points out most research has focused on dissatisfaction with weight, wanting to be thinner and although recent work is focusing more on boys and men, the subject of most body image research in the last 30 years has been young women (Tiggemann, 2004). These good or bad feelings are influenced by the media, who we see on TV, in movies, in magazines, and on social media. However, we can make conscious decisions about what we read, watch and google boogle so we are not totally powerless, as we can change.

One person's pain is another person's profit. The Cosmetic Surgery Solicitors survey of 789 British adults gives a sense of how people feel about the way they look, including the vital question: "Do you love your nose? This became current in August 2023 with debates about how Bradley Cooper, put on Bernstein's nose when he made a film about him. The great conductor had a large hooter.

Of those polled by Cosmetic, 52 per cent lack confidence in their own appearance to some degree. Only 6 per cent say they are "extremely confident" about it – the total narcissists perhaps. There are gender differences. More than 60 per cent of men are confident about their appearance to some degree, while only 44 per cent of women are. A total of 39 per cent said they "rarely" like their appearance in photographs taken by other people, while 20 per cent said they never do. Only 2 per cent said they always like how they appear in other people's photos. When it comes to selfies, 31 per cent only "rarely" like how they look in these pictures, and 20 per cent never like that, while only 3 per cent always indulge in self-adoration. A total of 25 per cent of those polled tend to avoid taking selfies, and 17 per cent avoid doing so at all costs.

When asked "Do you love your nose?" most are fairly positive. The most common rating was 7/10, with 18 per cent of respondents voting this way. Just over 40 per cent said they liked or loved it, while 37 per cent seemed not to care if they had a horrible hooter. A total of 70% would not consider having cosmetic surgery on their noses, compared to only 16 per cent who were thinking about it. The cosmetic surgery business is thriving, nevertheless. A personal note – my father's mother had a huge nose which looked much like a bulb of garlic. I still loved her. The fact that Jews supposedly have huge noses has been a feature of anti-semitism and Nazi propaganda cartoons revelled in the enormous Yiddish hooter.

The Savvy Psychologist

Cultures influence our affective body image. Monica Johnson, who calls herself the Savvy Psychologist, says she is Black, "and the idealisation of large backsides is a part of my culture. Guess who doesn't have a large butt. Me. But this doesn't make me any less Black or my body image any less positive. I welcome the Bulgarian Squats that my trainer recommends, hoping I'll get slightly more rotund glutes, but I know I'll never be on the same level as Megan Thee Stallion."

(Megan Thee is an American rapper).

"And this does not change my value as a person."

A negative body image shows in many ways. You don't buy new clothes; you don't look in mirrors. You hide your legs under long pants because you have thicker thighs. The message is that your body is bad. The Savvy Psychologist, wrote in Psychology Today, "The first time I wore a two-piece swimsuit, I was close to 400 pounds. I was inspired by Gabifresh, who had dropped on the scene as a fashion blogger and eventually started her own (larger person) swimsuit line. It was liberating to let it all hang out. We are four-dimensional beings and it's okay if our curves reflect that."

The psychologist is savvy indeed. "You can be dissatisfied with something and still accept it. If you're going to compare your body to other peoples', at least find comparisons that make you feel included and not ones that make you feel ostracised." So don't compare yourself to supermodels. This advice reminds me of George Mikes, a brilliant humourist and author of How to be an Alien, who told me once that we can all find something we are better at than others. I may not look as handsome as George Clooney, but can he say "Good morning" in Turkish?

3. Cognitive

These are the thoughts and beliefs that you hold about your body. For example, you might think, "if I build muscle in my chest and arms, I'll feel better about myself." Plenty of media offers help. *Iron Man Magazine* was founded in 1936. The magazine has always stressed the health and character-building aspects of weight-training. It is published in Japan, Australia, Sweden, Norway, and Italy.

Some iron history. Arnold Schwarzenegger began lifting weights at the age of 15 and went on to win the Mr. Universe title at age 20 and subsequently won the Mr. Olympia title seven times. He was one of the greatest bodybuilders of all time. He did not reply to my e mail asking for an interview. In the spirit of Johnny Weissmuller, who was a champion swimmer and then starred as Tarzan, Arnie moved into the movies and became a Hollywood action star, with his breakthrough in the sword and sorcery epic *Conan the Barbarian* (1982) who had no problems with his body image. Just like James Bond. Arnie then became Governor of California and would have had a chance to reach the White House if the American constitution did not insist Presidents had to be born in the US.

Despite the name Iron Man, women have also become interested in muscle building. The Savvy Psychologist reflects:

> "Maybe you're a woman in her 30s who is upset about face and body wrinkles and thinks, "If I can just maintain how I look now, I'll be happy."

If/then contingencies like this often add up to maybe/never results. If you inherently dislike yourself, you'll move the goal post. You'll gain

20 pounds of muscle and then say, "I just need to gain 10 more." Many people change their bodies but are never mentally satisfied. There is always a little more weight to lose, a few more wrinkles to smooth out, and a stomach roll that shows up that wasn't there before.

Be realistic with yourself about your goals and your potential, Savvy suggests. Instead of trying to avoid aging altogether, perhaps you should define for yourself what aging gracefully looks like. Advertising is helping. The cosmetic company Dove now uses older and larger women in their promotional material.

4. Behavioural

The last aspect of body image is behavioural. These are the actions you take in relation to your body image. According to the National Eating Disorders Collaboration, when a person is dissatisfied with the way they look, they may isolate themselves or employ unhealthy behaviours as a means to change appearance.

During the early 2000's researchers agreed that body image disturbance is a multidimensional symptom of various components associated with body image. More recently, researchers have increasingly looked at anorexia as a biologically based mental disorder, like schizophrenia.

According to Disorders in Social Relationships published by the Sciences Po University Press, anorexia nervosa usually affects middle- and upper-class girls.

The National Eating Disorders Association estimates that between 0.3 and 0.4 per cent of young women and 0.1 per cent of young men suffer from anorexia. They argue that approximately 1 per cent of women and 0.3 per cent of men reported anorexia during their lifetimes, according to the 2020 Breakthrough Research in Anorexia Nervosa by Drs. Cynthia Bulik and Walter Kaye.

Between the ages of 15–24 women who suffer from anorexia are at a 10 per cent greater risk of dying than others at the same age. A 2020 review found that anorexia runs in families and is often fatal.

I believe there is a fifth component to body image and one way to introduce it is with a quote from Goethe, Freud's favourite writer.

Know thyself. 'If I knew myself, I'd run away,' Goethe wrote. He would never have lain on the analytic couch. My firth component to body image is the unconscious view. Body image is also subjective. Do we know everything about what we feel about our bodies? We should not assume that what we see of ourselves is the entire picture.

Wittgenstein wrote that of what we cannot speak we must stay silent and the often-silent unconscious has its own rumbles, desires and fears.

The dangers of a negative body image

A negative body image can make you abusive – to yourself. Do you call yourself names, or starve yourself, or exercise to the point of exhaustion?

Susie Orbach's *Fat is a Feminist Issue* is a classic. In the book, she suggests that even though girls know that the bodies idealised in the media aren't real and they have physically been altered by surgery or digital manipulation, it doesn't alter the fact that, "The deluge of images that wallpapers our world has seeped into all of our consciousnesses. It has changed the way we view our bodies and what we can and should do to our bodies, including those of our children. Without a body that girls feel all right about, nothing much in their lives feels OK. Their bodies cause them trouble and worry. All the normal difficulties of growing up, dealing with the conflicts, choices and angsts of adolescence, get subsumed under a preoccupation to get one's body right."

Orbach argues, "preoccupation with how the body appears has become a crucial aspect of female experience." And it can affect the behaviour of girls as young as five years old who want to copy the popstars they see on screen. This can also affect girls' behaviour towards food and dieting as the media portrays a certain slim body image as ideal. Orbach goes on to say:

"Dieting is even more popular than it was when Fat Is A Feminist Issue was first published 28 years ago. Eating has become a psychological, moral, medical, aesthetic and cultural statement...Thin is wise; fat is bad." Orbach adds; "This mindset, this sense that one is too large or too fat, has penetrated into our awareness so that girls and women, boys and men, become increasingly self-conscious of their body size."

Science has fuelled these obsessions. In the 1830s Adolphe Jacques Quetelet, a Belgian sociologist, astronomer, and mathematician who tutored Victoria's husband Prince Albert was searching for a way to relate an individual's height to their ideal weight as a tool for studying populations. In 1972 his ideas inspired the creation of the Body Mass Index, which is a measure of whether you're a healthy weight for your height. For most adults, the healthy weight range is indicated by a BMI score of 18.5 to 24.9. However, according to the NHS website, the BMI score "has some limitations because it measures whether a person is carrying too much weight but not too much fat. For example, people who are very muscular, like professional sportspeople, can have a high BMI without much fat."

Furthermore, Orbach argues that that "fitness, not fat, determines our mortality. You can be fat, fit and healthy. Body fascism and the tyranny of thin and the sense that we should all be one size is not only unrealistic, it is unhealthy and unattainable."

However, even if we know this to be true, it is difficult to detach from a wish to conform to the ideal body shape that is portrayed constantly in the media. We might not even consciously realise the impact that such visual imagery is having on us.

As Orbach points out, "In 1995 TV was first introduced to Fiji showing many imported US shows. Only three years later, 11.9 per cent of the teenage girls were suffering with bulimia, a previously unknown behaviour. This shocking fact reverberates in my mind when I try to understand the growth of eating and body image problems today and the factors that have accelerated them globally. It is not only key for the young women of Fiji, but also for young women in England, Ireland, Scotland, Wales, Europe, North and South America, and increasingly those countries brought into globalism."

Body image is inextricably bound up with issues of self-esteem, and self-worth. Sadly, statistics reported by Stem 4, a charity that supports teenagers with mental health issues, show that 77 per cent of teenage girls today worry about their body image – which has led to some tragedies – and an increasing number of boys worry too.

The power of body image

The power of body image is significant. We see this through history in the depiction the ideal body image in painting and sculpture. Elizabeth I was well aware of the value of projecting her looks and, of course, no one dared paint an unflattering portrait. Parliament Square glories in many statues of the powerful, including Winston Churchill and William Gladstone. Churchill hated the painting that the Commons commissioned for his 80th birthday, and it has disappeared since then. The late Queen Elizabeth was far too polite to ever criticise any of her many portraits. This book deals with the perceived images of many celebrities and famous figures like Queen Elizabeth I, Roosevelt, and Coco Chanel. It is safe to say they were all more than a little vain. Vanity is not to be avoided in dealing with body image.

The vanity of psychology and the psychology of vanity

Vanity is part of what makes us human. If it were not for our vanity, the billion-dollar cosmetics industry would not exist. Would fashion ever be in fashion? But there is a counterpoint to the lament of vanity.

Benjamin Franklin recognized the unappealing reputation of vanity. However, when writing to his son explaining why he agreed to write his life story, he admitted the task might "gratify" his vanity. He wrote; most people dislike vanity in others, whatever share they have of it themselves; but I give it fair quarter wherever I meet with it, being persuaded that it is often productive of good to the possessor, and to others that are within his sphere of action; and therefore, in many cases, it would not be altogether absurd if a man were to thank God for his vanity among the other comforts of life."

All is vanity, says the Bible, but Franklin seems to be suggesting that is not the whole truth. Vanity, however unappealing it is in exaggerated forms, may stimulate some of the remarkable things that we create – even though we may be appear vain when we reflect on them. Yes, vanity is something to be thankful for. It has driven many women and men to some remarkable achievements, he argued.

The criminal look

If the ideal body image has power over us, what about the flipside? In his famous story The Murders in the Rue Morgue, Edgar Allen Poe made the murderer an orangutan, which may have influenced the 19th-century Italian criminologist Cesare Lombroso, who needed his head examined, it could be said.

He argued that the "born criminal" could be identified by such items as a sloping forehead, ears of unusual size, asymmetry of the face, prognathism, excessive length of arms, asymmetry of the cranium, and other "physical stigmata." Thieves, rapists, and murderers could be distinguished by specific characteristics, he believed. He has left a nasty legacy. Police profiling of suspicious individual has caused much controversy. According to Lombroso's theory, Charles III is suspect as he has long ears, but our new King has no criminal record.

The opposite of Lombroso's criminals are those whose faces show the Golden Ratio like Bella Hadid, who is said to be the most beautiful woman on earth (see Chapter 2 for more on the Golden Ratio). How we see ourselves is psychologically important, but what makes us feel the way we do about our bodies? If you are a narcissist, are you to blame? Did your mother say to you, 'You're so handsome' every day" petting you like her little lamb? Or did your brother or sister say to you 'you look like porridge, yuck?' leaving you with a life-long inferiority complex?

What influences our body image?

The consensus among psychologists is that self-esteem, gender, media messages, and pressure or support from peers and family influence body image, as well as how one reacts to the experience of our bodies. One example – girls who feel they are heavier tend to have lower self-esteem, and those with lower self-esteem are increasingly likely to say they are unhappy with their body size or shape, regardless of age or gender. How much of our self-concept does our body image represent? One finding is that teenagers who do sports have a better body image, but the association is small. (Mendo et al., 2017). No one knows how stable or extensive the link is and it will differ from individual to individual. A cynic might suggest power also matters. It is unlikely that any dictator has been told he is not physically perfect.

Culture is not static. Once, for example, it was thought good to be fat as that showed you were not poor. For much of the last 50 years, however, to be fat was seen as unattractive. Think of the nicknames like podge. I was podgy at school and was called heffalump. I was lucky that in the 1960s social media did not exist so I did not have to bear the humiliation of having my podginess broadcast to the whole world which would have happened today when 10 million new photographs are uploaded to Facebook every hour. First, social media users themselves often present an idealised version of themselves uploading only the most attractive images of themselves. Second, social media is generally used to interact with one's peers and research suggests that how you compare your appearance to and with peers may be particularly influential for how you see yourself. Third, social media revels in cruel comments and has led to tragedies like that of the teenager Molly Russell who killed herself because she saw her 'friends' on Facebook were so vile about her.

To begin at the beginning.

When do children develop a body image?

The great French psychologist Jean Piaget in his observations with his wife noted the stages of development of their three children. He wrote that the child lived in the present, but he never spoke of body image. (It is interesting that Piaget studied psychoanalysis and even tried to psychoanalyse his mother who put up with her son's cheek for a year and then stopped her analysis).

It is clear that notions of body image, body image ideals and body dissatisfaction develop much earlier than was once thought. Psychologists now see children as young as six who have body image problems. Smolak (2004, pp. 19–20) asserts, "We know little about the development of body image, particularly during the pre-school and early elementary school years." Body dissatisfaction is especially prevalent among children who are overweight (Kelly et al., 2011; Puhl & Latner, 2007; Ricciardelli & McCabe, 2001) estimated that between 60 per cent and 99 per cent of children and adolescents with overweight/obesity want a smaller body size. Fat children also report higher levels of body dissatisfaction compared to non-overweight peers (Gouveia, Frontini, Canavarro, & Moreira, 2014).

Birkbeck and Drummond (2003) in a study on body image and the pre-pubescent child, studied forty-seven children (25 male; 22 female) aged between five and six years were interviewed three times over 12 months. The interviews revealed being fat was seen as negative. One of their subjects was Jenna; her interviews highlight the plight of many younger children particularly with older siblings. At the time of the first interview Jenna was aged five years, four months. Here is what she had to say over the 12-month period. When she chose a lower number figure, Jenna was asked: I: Why do you want to be this one? J: Because it is skinny. I: Why do you think you would like to be skinny? J: Because my brother always calls me fat. I: What do you think of that? J: I don't like it.

At the second interview, Jenna was six years, zero months old and chose an even smaller image. She claimed: J: My brother always teases me; saying I am fat: and how does that make you feel? J: Bad. I: Do they say it in a bad way? J: Yes. I: Do you think you are fat? J: No. When I get really angry with them, I scream at them. It is not funny because I don't think I am fat. Sometimes I cry.

At the third interview Jenna was six years, four months old. She once again chose her ideal body figure as being the smallest. Upon reflection she commented: J: Because it is skinny. I: Do you think you are skinny? J: No, I think I look like this one. She chose a thin one. Why would you like that one? J: So, my brother will not tease me anymore. I: What do your brothers do? J: They tease me and say, "you're fat!" I: Why do you think they do that? J: I don't know, they are just mean. I: So, what would happen if you were image 1? J: They would stop teasing me. I: Do you think they might tease you about being very skinny? J: No, they wouldn't do that.

For the boys, the ideal image was often larger than their perceived real image. Larger bodies were seen as more capable or more useful than smaller bodies, which is consistent with the literature (Drummond & Philips, 2001; Drummond, 2003). James (six years, one month), for example, said, "I want to be this one because it is bigger." Furthermore, he identified that "I would be able to kick higher."

We need to understand why body image dissatisfaction has become so common in Western society and starts so young. The past two decades have seen more body image research with younger and younger children. (Smolak, 2004). There are anecdotes of children as young as seven years of age eating less (Kostanski & Gullone, 1995). Tiggemann (2001) concluded that body image dissatisfaction could be identified in children as young as six years of age. He noted that "six- and seven-year-old girls rated their ideal as significantly thinner in a way that five-year-old girls did not." The results of this study suggest that significant developments in girls' perception of body image may occur between five and six years. One in four children aged between seven and ten years old has dieted to lose weight. These statistics represent a compelling reason to understand more about how children younger than seven years of age develop their perceptions of their own body and the bodies of other people. Those studies that have been performed suggest children between five and six years of age have some notion of how society disapproves of what I call podgitude.

2 Body Image Ideals through the Ages

The Dream of a perfect body and body image

Did our ancestors bother with how they looked? Yes. Time travel to 10,000 BCE. Cavepersons started to use sharp rocks, shells or flint to scrape hair from their face and head.

For the ancient Greeks a beautiful body was proof of a wonderful mind. The word they used to describe someone as beautiful was *kaloskagathos,* which derives from the adjective καλός ("beautiful") and αγαθός ("good" or "virtuous") which combines physical and spiritual beauty into one harmonious ensemble.

Survival of a city depended on having physically strong, resilient citizen soldiers so cities encouraged fitness in great sporting and religious festivals including the Olympic games.

The first Olympics were held around 776 BCE and initially consisted of religious festivities to honour Zeus. The games eventually included foot races, horse races, wrestling, boxing, pankration (a type of mixed martial art), chariot races, and the ancient pentathlon – running, jumping, wrestling, and throwing the javelin and discus – which is much like the modern pentathlon, apart from the wrestling.

The city of Sparta produced disciplined warriors who could subdue its slaves and put the fear of the Greek gods in its political rivals. When Philip II of Macedon was expanding his control over Greece in 346 BCE, he demanded the Spartans surrender and warned, "If I bring my forces into your land, I will ravage your homesteads, massacre your people, and destroy your city." The Spartans warned him off with one word: "*If.*"

By their pots you shall know them. Much Greek pottery was decorated with male figures performing various exercises, although no one seems to have found one which shows men touching their toes.

DOI: 10.4324/9781003425878-2

Unlike most Greek cities Sparta trained its women. Girls had to be fit so they could bear children for the Spartan state. Girls were well fed, were encouraged to exercise, play sports, and to stay physically active throughout life. And to dance even.

Some modern writers have used Spartan principles to develop contemporary exercises. I quote the following from Classical Wisdom – and some of it is wonderfully odd.

> "You will need a large open field, preferably with an oval or circular track at the perimeter, a frisbee or other throwing disk, and a weighted object you can grasp with both hands (like a kettle bell). At one side of the field, place your throwing disk, on the other side of the field place your kettle bell or other weight."

Classical Wisdom recommends listening to audiobooks, so while you run or throw the discus you can listen to the *Iliad* or any of the myths of Theseus or Heracles. While listening, jog at a moderate pace around the perimeter of the field and ponder the crucial lessons you are hearing.

The Greeks were more physically active than most of us today. One of the puzzles is why the Greeks did not invent the bicycle. They knew how to work metal after all.

For Aristotle, beauty was an objectively real quality. He was so dazzled by beauty he argued that in some cases a handsome man with no other qualities could outclass/beat another less handsome person with more qualifications. Socrates believed that a beautiful man would suffer so, while beauty is admired, it is also to be feared.

Ovid

Appearance matters in Ovid's Amores (Loves), I.14 when the narrator chides his girlfriend Corinna when her hair falls out after a bad dye job. He wrote:

> "Stop dyeing your hair.
> Now you have no hair left to tint.
> And what could be longer than your hair, if only you had let it alone? It fell all the way down to your hips…
> …It was neither dark nor gold
> but, though it was neither colour, every colour was mixed, like the colour the tall cedar has in the wet valleys
> of hilly Ida when the bark is stripped.

> Add that hair was docile and fitted to a hundred styles and never a cause of grief."

Medieval ideas of beauty were contradictory. Physical beauty was a sign of high moral virtue. Yet beautiful women were potentially dangerous, as they could lead men into sin. And woe betide women who used ointments as beauty was a gift of God, so trying to make yourself looked better showed pride, one of the deadly sins which could make a girl cosy up to Lucifer.

There were 30 standards of beauty and the number three was key. "Three to be long — hands, legs, and hair; three to be white, three to be pink, three to be round, three to be narrow, and so on." said Arthur Marwick, in his book *Beauty in History* (London: Thames & Hudson, 1988). The beautiful maiden had well-shaped bright white shins and smooth thighs, carefully arranged golden blonde tresses, smooth, tender white shoulders, dark black eyebrows, and radiant skin.

In 1995 Claudio Da Soller of the University of Missouri detailed the medieval European archetype of beauty: "a small head; blond hair; eyebrows set apart, long and arched; a narrow chin; large, prominent, colourful, and shining eyes, with long lashes; small, delicate ears; a long throat; a finely chiselled nose; small, even, sharp and white teeth, close together; red gums; red lips finely drawn; a small mouth; and her face white, hairless, bright and smooth." These features are "baby-like," seen in the large eyes, small hips, smooth skin, white teeth, small ears, and a slender nose.

The *Trotula*, a medieval text for women written in the 12th century, includes recipes and instructions that help women clear up their skin, colour their hair and even get rid of the stench from their mouths. Medieval toothpaste was not much use. Some excerpts from the *Trotula* offer medieval beauty tips!

Beautiful hair

"After leaving the bath, let her adorn her hair, and first of all let her wash it with a cleanser such as this. Take the ashes of burnt vine, the chaff of barley nodes, and liquorice wood (so that it may the more brightly shine), and sowbread; boil the chaff and the sowbread in water.

With the chaff and the ash and the sowbread, let a pot having at its base two or three small openings be filled. Let the water in which the sowbread and the chaff were previously cooked be poured into the pot, so that it is strained by the small openings. With this cleanser let the woman wash her head. After the washing, let her leave it to dry by itself, and her hair will be golden and shimmering." it stated

> "Also, noblewomen should wear musk in their hair, or clove, or both, but take care that it not be seen by anyone. Also, the veil, with which the head is tied should be put on with cloves and musk, nutmeg, and other sweet-smelling substances."

Poetry is again useful. Gwerful Mechain was a daring Welsh-language poet. In her ode to pubic hair, she criticizes men for praising the other parts of a woman's body, but not the genitalia. She urges poets to "let songs about the quim circulate," and ends by saying "lovely bush, God save it."

Her most famous poem is: "Cywydd y cedor." Or, to non-Welsh speakers, "Poem to the vagina." "Vulva" would be a more accurate translation. "I rejected that because [it] for me at least, has a slightly clinical ring to it," the critic Katie Gramich says. Other translations have taken a different tack; Jon Stone calls it, simply, "Cunt," while Dafydd Johnston buttoned it right back up again with the precise but hardly erotic, "The Female Genitals."

It is a masterful piece of writing, which Katie Gramich believes "shows off her skill at 'dyfalu' thinking up ingenious metaphors to describe something) extremely well." For my part, "Poem to the vagina" provides a holistic introduction to Mechain's poetic approach; not only is it thought to be a retort to male contemporaries (specifically, Dafydd ap Gwilym's "Poem to the penis"), the more liberal of Gramich's translations, demonstrates how it overtly engages and celebrates "you female body, you're strong and fair / A faultless fleshy court plumed with hair," while also expressing a general disdain for men's opinions. In frustration that will be familiar to so many people with vaginas, Mechain bemoans men for "ignoring the best bit, silly sod ... The place I love, the place I bless / The hidden quim beneath the dress." Quite.

The Virgin Queen

In Elizabethan times, the wealthy were very hair-conscious and spent much time and money getting their hair dyed red or blond. The perfect woman had snow-white skin and red cheeks and lips.

At different periods of Queen Elizabeth I's life, her subjects saw her differently. It was very much a case of "beauty is in the eye of the beholder." To those who worshipped Elizabeth as Gloriana, she does appear eternally youthful, while foreigners were more objective, indifferent, and described what they saw:

> "Her face is comely rather than handsome, but she is tall and well-formed, with good skin, though swarthy; she has fine eyes."
>
> Venetian Ambassador, Giovanni Michiele, 1557

Sir James Melville in his Memoirs described the young Queen's hair as "more reddish than yellow, and curled in appearance naturally."

> "...her face oblong, fair, but wrinkled, her eyes small, yet black and pleasant; her nose a little hooked, her lips narrow and her teeth black; her hair was of an auburn colour, but false; upon her head she had a small crown. Her bosom was uncovered, as all the English ladies have it till they marry. Her hands were slender, her fingers rather long, and her stature neither tall nor low; her air was stately, and her manner of speaking mild and obliging."

Paul Hentzner, German visitor to Greenwich Palace, 1598.
Sir Francis Bacon described her as "tall of stature":

> "Slender and straight; her hair inclined to pale yellow; her forehead large and fair; her eyes lively and sweet, but short sighted, her nose somewhat rising in the midst; her countenance was somewhat long, but yet of admirable beauty, in a most delightful composition of majesty and modesty."
>
> Sir John Hayward

> "Very youthful still in appearance, seeming no more than twenty years of age."
>
> Thomas Platter, 1599

In her speech at Tilbury in 1588 as the Spanish Armada was approaching, Elizabeth made her appearance critical. Different descriptions of her outfit exist, but there is consensus that she wore a plumed helmet and a steel cuirass over a white velvet gown to depict herself as a warrior. Her words were also fierce. She said she might have the body of a woman, but she had the heart of a king.

A high forehead was considered very attractive, so women shaved the hair from their front hairlines. There were two main styles: the "padded" style and the "frizzed" style, both worn by the Queen. The first one had to be done with two pieces called "rats" – they looked like them - and framed the face with a heart-shape form. The second one was a curly and rather casual hairdo. Trendy Elizabethan women wore hairnets ("cauls"), or hats called "coifs." Hat makers thrived as they frilled up hats with feathers, pearls, glass jewels, spangles, gold thread, embroidery, and lace.

As we saw with Gwerful Mechain, the body beautiful has always been adored in art and poetry. John Donne was Dean of St Paul's at the start of the 17th century, and unusual among clerics as he praised the body as much as the soul. Here's an extract from one of my favourite poems:

To His Mistress Going to Bed

Off with that girdle, like heaven's Zone glistering,
But a far fairer world encompassing.
Unpin that spangled breastplate which you wear,
That th'eyes of busy fools may be stopped there.
Unlace yourself, for that harmonious chime,
Tells me from you, that now it is bedtime.
Off with that happy busk, which I envy,
That still can be, and still can stand so nigh.
Your gown going off, such beauteous state reveals,
As when from flowery meads th'hill's shadow steals.

Beauty is not just in the eye of the beholder but in his or her culture too.

During the French revolution of 1789, short hair became extremely popular for both men and women to make the point they were not hated aristocrats. At the same time rabbis debated the issue of hair. Our images of Jehovah incidentally usually show him as an old man with flowing locks and a beard. Some rabbis were for wigs while others were against them, claiming that a wig fashioned from human hair did not pass muster as a hair covering. In the introduction, I promised a light interlude with a Rabbi and his wife. We now time travel back to Chez Rabbi where the rabbi and his wife are sitting down to dinner. The wife removes her wig:

WIFE: You can't wear this in the desert. It itches like mad and worse when you kiss me.

RABBI: If I'd known how fussy you were I'd have married your sister.
WIFE: A husband is supposed to love his wife.
RABBI: That's for Christians.
WIFE: You can have this for your dinner then.
(She cuts some of the hair from the wig and mixes it into his kosher stew.)

Some rabbis were anti wig. The Hatam Sofer (1762–1839), one of the leading rabbis of the 19th century, forbade the women in his family to wear wigs even after he died. Most rabbis, however, accepted wigs as sufficient hair coverings for women.

A brief history of corsets

The term "corset" was in use in the late 14th century, from the French "corset" which meant "a kind of laced bodice." Its meaning as a "stiff supporting so constricting undergarment for the waist, worn chiefly by women to shape the figure" dates from 1795.

The main purpose of 18th-century stays was to raise and shape the breasts, tighten the midriff, support the back, improve posture to help a woman stand straight, with the shoulders down and back, and only slightly narrow the waist, creating a "V" shaped upper torso over which the outer garment would be worn.

By the 1830s steel stays had begun to replace the classic whalebone. The diarist Emily Eden said she had to obtain a silver "husk" before sailing with her brother to India because a humid climate rusted the usual steel. Corsets and the Raj would make a good PhD subject.

For dress reformists of the late 1800s, corsets were a dangerous moral 'evil', promoting promiscuous views of female bodies. Corsets were also seen as a health risk as they could remove ribs or rearrange internal organs and compromise fertility. Preachers inveighed against tightlacing; doctors counselled patients against it.

American women active in the anti-slavery and temperance movements, demanded sensible clothing that would not restrict their movement.

In 1873 Elizabeth Stuart Phelps Ward wrote:

> Burn up the corsets! ... No, nor do you save the whalebones, you will never need whalebones again. Make a bonfire of the cruel steels that have lorded it over your thorax and abdomens for so

many years and heave a sigh of relief, for your emancipation I assure you, from this moment has begun.

But corsets still sold well. Edward VII, when he was Prince of Wales, was not a fan as it made undressing his lovers such hard work. For years he had an affair with Winston Churchill's mother. He was a lazy lover and sent her a postcard once asking her to wear the kimono which slipped off easily so he could slip in.

Soon after the United States' entry into the First World War in 1917, the U.S. War Industries Board asked women to stop buying corsets to free up metal for war production. This liberated some 28,000 tons of metal, enough to build two battleships. In 1968 protesters threw a number of feminine products into a "Freedom Trash Can." These included girdles and corsets, which the protesters called "instruments of female torture."

Playtex still sell girdles and Madonna's ironic underwear worn outside the body shows some kind of fetish corset still has power.

I have not dealt with transgender and body image because the subject is so fluid, but it would be wrong to imagine this is a modern phenomenon as the life of Charles d'Éon (1728–1810) illustrates. I first learned of him in T.H. White's wonderful *The Age of Scandal* and d'Éon was certainly a scandal. S/he was a French diplomat, spy, and soldier. S/he (which seems the right way to pronoun d'Éon) fought in the Seven Years' War and spied for France while in Russia and England. S/he had androgynous physical characteristics and natural abilities as a mimic and appeared publicly as a man and pursued masculine occupations for 49 years, while appearing at the court of Empress Elizabeth of Russia as a woman. Starting in 1777, d'Éon lived as a woman and was officially recognised as a woman by King Louis XVI. There is even a Soviet novel about him, *By Plume and Sword*, written by Valentin Pikul in 1963 and first published in 1972.

Most of what is known about d'Éon's early life comes from a partly ghost-written autobiography, *The Interests of the Chevalier d'Éon de Beaumont* and Bram Stoker's essay on the Chevalier in his 1910 book *Famous Impostors*.

Some physiology. D'Éon claimed to have been assigned female at birth but was brought up as a boy because Louis d'Éon de Beaumont could only inherit from his in-laws if he had a son. He became a writer and got noticed through two works on financial and administrative questions published in 1753. D'Éon served as a secretary to the administrator of the fiscal department, and was appointed a royal censor for history and literature in 1758.

Five years later he/she became chargé d'affaires in April 1763 in London where he also doubled as a spy for the French king. D'Éon formed connections with English nobility by sending them bottles of d'Éon's vineyard in France. Claret makes friends.

Being binary did not stop D'Éon becoming a Freemason in 1768. Although d'Éon habitually wore a dragoon's uniform, rumours circulated in London that d'Éon was actually a woman. And city gents bet on her or his true gender. D'Éon was invited to join, but declined, saying that an examination would be dishonouring, whatever the result.

After the death of Louis XV in 1774, d'Éon tried to negotiate a return from exile. The writer Pierre de Beaumarchais who is famous for The Barber of Seville and the Marriage of Figaro represented the French government in the negotiations. The resulting twenty-page treaty permitted d'Éon to return to France and retain a pension but required that d'Éon turn over the correspondence relating to his spying.

Madame Campan writes in her memoirs: "This eccentric being had long solicited permission to return to France; but it was necessary to find a way of sparing the family he had offended the insult they would see in his return; he was therefore made to resume the costume of that sex to which in France everything is pardoned. The desire to see his native land once more determined him to submit to the condition, but he revenged himself by combining the long train of his gown and the three deep ruffles on his sleeves with the attitude and conversation of a grenadier, which made him very disagreeable company."

King Louis XVI and his court complied with this demand but required in turn that d'Éon dress appropriately in women's clothing, although d'Éon was allowed to continue to wear the insignia of the Order of Saint-Louis. When the king's offer included funds for a new wardrobe of women's clothes, d'Éon agreed. After fourteen months of negotiation, d'Éon returned to France.

The surgeon who examined d'Éon's body said in the post-mortem certificate that the Chevalier had "male organs in every respect perfectly formed," while at the same time displaying feminine characteristics. A couple of characteristics described in the certificate were "unusual roundness in the formation of limbs," as well as "breast remarkably full."

D'Éon's body was buried in the churchyard of St Pancras Old Church, and d'Éon's remaining possessions were sold by Christie's in 1813. D'Éon's grave is listed on the Burdett-Coutts Memorial there as one of the important graves lost.

Some modern scholars have interpreted d'Éon as transgender. Havelock Ellis coined the term *eonism* to describe similar cases of transgender behaviour. It is rarely used now.

D'Eon's life seems to have influenced Virginia Woolf's novel Orlando about a hero who changed gender. And on April 15, 2024 *The Times* carried an interview with Britain's first transgender judge who complains of the way trans people are treated.

The Victorians

Queen Victoria felt makeup belonged on the stage with actresses and prostitutes, but that did not mean that her subjects stopped wearing makeup. They just got better at hiding it. Everything had to look natural. It was believed that cheeks painted with blush had to look flushed, and lips had to look bitten rather than painted. Eyebrows were lightly plucked and darkened with natural ingredients, and eyeliner all but disappeared in the Victorian era. Perfume was considered suitable, but only in floral scents and never applied directly to the skin.

Some Victorian women nibbled on wafers made of deadly arsenic to get bright eyes and a translucent complexion. They also put drops of belladonna, or deadly nightshade in their eyes to dilate their pupils and make their eyes look bigger. Never mind that belladonna in high concentration can cause blindness. A cheaper alternative was lemon or orange juice – imagine squirting that into your eye!

Pimples, freckles, and blemishes were considered shameful. White, blue, and pink powders could hide these blemishes or counteract the yellow glow of candlelight. Some businesses had secret back doors for their wealthy female clients so high society would never guess what they put on their faces.

Cold creams were the only cosmetic that a woman could be seen to use. Cosmetic companies touted cleansing creams made from very natural ingredients, intending to fight blemishes before they appeared.

Isabella Beeton remains famous today because her book on household management has been a best seller for 150 years. She was an excellent researcher – her book covers among much else how the Egyptian cooked and the symbolic value of cucumbers. She would no more neglect hair than neglect mayonnaise – and there is a connection.

She and her husband Samuel founded a magazine and hair was a topic. She discussed hair that had been "frizzed very much," and necklaces, French canes and even fashion hotspots. "For evening dinner, hair ought to be dressed in four rolls either side and finished off behind with a Marie Antoinette chignon, frizzed very much." Mrs Beeton also had this to say about hairdressing. "Hairdressing: is one of the most important parts of the lady's-maid's office. Lessons in hairdressing may be obtained, and at not an unreasonable charge, and a lady's-maid should initiate herself in the mysteries of hair-dressing before entering on her duties. If a mistress finds her maid handy, and willing to learn, she will not mind the expense of a few lessons, which are almost necessary, as the fashion and mode of dressing the hair is continually changing. Brushes and combs should be kept scrupulously clean, by washing them about twice a week; to do this oftener spoils the brushes, as very frequent washing makes them so very soft.

Hair had to be clean, Mrs. Beeton added.

Beeton died tragically young giving birth to her fourth child. But she and her husband had started a trend which became influential.

In the Edwardian era, magazines carried makeup adverts and skin-care advice, but women would still buy their makeup secretly. Pale skin remained popular until the First World War, but blonde hair was no longer the ideal, so women used henna to dye their hair in copper shades.

Charles Gibson's photographs of his Gibson Girls perpetuated the Edwardian ideal of beauty – brunettes with pencilled eyebrows, big hair, and tinted lips. Cheeks needed a healthy flush, but women still used belladonna in their eyes! Skincare also remained important, with women applying several creams during the day.

The glamorous movie stars of the 1930s finally brought cosmetics into the mass market, where they were sold in department stores. Two women Chanel and Colette were key figures.

In June 1932 a beauty salon opened in the Eighth Arrondissement of Paris. Its Art Deco interior evoked a medical clinic – albeit a very chic one – and its glass counters displayed new lines of lipsticks, perfumes, and creams. At the grand opening, the public saw an extraordinary sight: the middle-aged beautician giving makeovers was the greatest prose stylist in France. The products bore her name, Colette. She said that she was launching the line to save women from the ravages of time: "I know so well what one ought to spread upon a terrified female face, so full of hope in its decline." Some critics say Colette actually made some of her clients look older so that she would look better compared to them.

Colette prized the body over the mind – as suggested by the title of Judith Thurman's biography, *Secrets of the Flesh* – and believed that focussing on the physical was essential to writing "like a woman, without anything moralistic or theoretical." Unusually for a woman of her time, Colette adhered to a regular workout regimen, and she was an early adopter of the face-lift, battling back time. In two of her most famous books, *Chéri*, from 1920, and *The End of Chéri*, from 1926 – time is the enemy.

Chanel's talents as a dress maker were first spotted by the Mother Superior of the orphanage she was put in. Chanel became a brilliant pioneering designer and freed women from the tyranny of too many layers of clothes. She said it is always better to be slightly underdressed.

Chanel was antisemitic, and that should never be forgotten when admiring her couture. Both she and Colette were contemporaries of the pioneer of body image.

Fashion

Fashion is an important way that we present ourselves, as Dearborn observed back in 1918 in *The Psychology of Clothing*. He stated "one's clothes are one of the important things that intervenes between the individual personality and his environment, and you understand that life itself in a sense is a reaction of an individual to his environment. As Webb, a psychologist at the University of Madison, puts it, "As a matter of fact, our artificial coverings have become so much a part of our life that one may perhaps be allowed to apply the methods of the naturalist to their consideration, and deal with them as if they were part and parcel of the creature which wears them… We might almost consider clothes as a vicarious or artificial skin, almost an extension of the individual's boundary, involving important relationships between the person and his environment, spiritual as much as material. And that is the reason, the deeply fundamental reason, why there is so much real science in the physiology and the psychology of clothing, subjective and objective, personally and socially and industrially."

We do not know when our ancestors first started wearing clothes and there is no literature on Neanderthal haute couture. Dearborn claims 'their main clothes were a ring through the nose and a patch of red paint on the forehead'.

Dress style

Sociologists have argued that fashion is a pursuit of class distinction or a sort of 'conspicuous consumption' (Simmel 1904; Bourdieu

1984; Veblen, 1899). In her book, *The Psychology of Fashion* Carolyn Mair (2018) argues that 'fashion became more accessible across socio-economic strata' in the twentieth century'. She also points out that people dress not just to 'look prosperous'. She explores the psychological functions of fashion, including 'self-enhancement', 'self-categorisation', 'self-expression' and the construction of social identity and emphasises the adverse influence of the ideal body image on young children. Pre schoolgirls are targeted in ads for snazzy, even sexy clothes.

You are what you wear. And we wear less and less. Compare the Victorian woman who could only go into the sea in a bathing machine with women in itsy bitsy tiny bikinis today. The key designers are Chanel who we met earlier who created the little black dress and Mary Quant who popularised the mini skirt. Wearing less is a sign of feminine empowerment.

The reader who wants details of how fashion changed could read a hugely entertaining History of Vogue by Georgina Howell.

Is your ratio golden? Or is it silver or dross?

Some standards of beauty have not changed through the ages. Since the 4th century BCE, mathematicians have tried to figure out the equations for perfection. This led to the development of a set of measurements that led in turn to the ratio 1: 1.618, which is now often called "The Golden Ratio." This ratio shows up all over the human body, for example the length of the arms and legs divided by the length of the torso. It seems to describe what proportions look best. Painters and sculptors have known about the golden ratio for a long time and have used it to make sculptures and artwork that look like the perfect human form.

The Vitruvian Man, which Leonardo da Vinci drew around 1490 showed how the human body was the main source of proportion in the Classical orders of architecture. Vitruvius said that the upper body should be about 3.75 times the size of the lower body. This is close to the golden ratio of 1:1.6.

Faces are about 1.618 times longer than they are wide.

The distance between the top of the nose and the centre of the lips is 1.618 times greater than the distance between the centre of the lips and the chin.

The cosmetic surgeon Julian De Silva compiled his list of top ten women by using the Golden Ratio theory. He based his list on a calculated measurement of the size and position of the eyes, eyebrows, nose, lips, chin and jaw. Among all women, Bella Hadid ranked highest, with a result of 94.35 per cent of symmetry.

3 The Academic Study of Body Image

The scientific literature on body image dates to the 1930s when two pioneers worked. The first was Paul F. Schilder, the son of a Jewish silk merchant. He got his doctorate in medicine in 1909 from the University of Vienna and, as a result of his work *Self-Esteem and Personality*, received his Doctor of Philosophy in 1917. The second pioneer was Françoise Dolto, who was called France's favourite granny by *Le Monde* when she died. The millions who listened to her weekly broadcast on national radio felt guided by her as parents, yet Dolto is curiously unknown in the English-speaking world.

In 1919 Schilder became a member of the Viennese Psychoanalytical Association. Freud clashed fiercely with Schilder. In March Freud wrote to his devoted follower Karl Abraham: "Today I received – after the Simmel – a monograph extracted from the *Lewandowskysche Sammlung* (notebook number 15): *Delusion and knowledge* by Paul Schilder (Leipzig), which, in its results, is already thoroughly analytical, and which only leaves aside, as is appropriate, the Oedipus complex. Of course, Schilder. acts as if these gentlemen had discovered everything themselves, or almost everything. In short, this is how German clinicians are going to 'appropriate' our discoveries. All things considered, I vow, it is of no importance."

Nine years later Schilder travelled to Baltimore where he became a guest lecturer at Johns Hopkins University. He later became clinical director of the psychiatric division of Bellevue Hospital in New York. In 1935 he published *The Image and Appearance of the Human Body*, which he thought was his most important book. He and Freud clashed over the question of training analyses. Freud wrote to him that those of the first analytic generation who weren't analysed did not boast of the fact, and that "whenever it was possible it was done: Jones and Ferenczi, for instance, had long analyses." Both those men

DOI: 10.4324/9781003425878-3

were crucial in the development of psychoanalysis. Schilder was never analysed himself which reinforced Freud's view that he should not be seen as an authority. Freud himself of course conducted his own self-analysis as he discovered the royal road to the unconscious, but then he was the creator of analysis.

Schilder liked to look dapper. He argued that everyone had a (potentially infinite) number of separate body-images. He also explored the role of changes in body image in schizophrenia – a common symptom is feeling disconnected from one's body.

There is now a learned journal devoted to the subject, *The Journal of Body Image*, and there are many tests of every aspect of the subject.

Françoise Dolto

Wittgenstein wrote that of what we cannot speak we must stay silent and that is relevant to the unconscious, which has its own rumbles, desires and fears. In *The Unconscious Body Image* (1984) French paediatrician and psychoanalyst Dolto described how unconsciously held mental images of the body and its functioning affect feelings and ideas of identity, and how emotions and ideas impact upon the body's functioning by way of these unconscious images. Dolto accepted Freud and claimed unconscious body images are generated at each stage of development (oral, anal, genital, latency, and puberty).

Dolto (1908–88) belonged to the second generation of French analysts. She was close to Jacques Lacan, the influential but sometimes hard to understand analyst for Anglo Saxons at least. She showed how parent-child interactions affect the development of the unconscious body image, which influences the functioning of the real body. She makes much of what she calls psychic castration at each developmental stage.

One of her cases was a restless eight-year-old Giles who was always looking around as if he were under threat. Dolto got him to draw, and his drawings were full of arrows whose target he was. Himself. He linked that with the word English which made sense. He had been evacuated from Paris in 1940 and the car he was in had an accident as his family were fleeing south. Then he nearly drowned when his father was teaching him to swim. After that he clung to his mother, literally taking refuge between her legs.

At what was meant to be their last session it became clear that taking refuge between his mother's legs was erotic. His restlessness was an attempt to cope with the anxieties provoked by the two accidents. Unfortunately, Dolto did not reveal if bringing all this out in words helped the child.

There are parallels between her work and that of D.W. Winnicott, the English analyst whose writings are always intelligible. He argued that one should help mothers tend to their baby, but if they found that hard that could not be done by lecturing them.

Winnicott was interested in the relationship between maternal care and the baby. The I of the mother boosts the baby whose self is weak, even non-existent. Winnicott uses the term *holding* for the care the mother gives the child and justifies it because the good enough mother – one of Winnicott's important phrases – holds the newborn well enough. Her or his centre of gravity is not in his own body but lies between his mother and him. For the child, holding is vital to build her or his sense of self.

If the baby is not held well psychically as well as physically she will suffer these feelings – that she or he is in bits, that he or she is falling with no end, dying, that there is no hope of re-establishing contact with the mother. Some mothers do not manage to hold their child and so need help. Some mothers find that hard especially if they feel they were themselves abandoned by their mother. That is the eternal question who mothered the mother?

Helping distressed mothers was not easy. Dolto referred to a case where a *surveillante*, a watchful nurse, did not more than just give advice. She added: "I have to say that personally I would never have dared do what this *surveillante* did. Psychoanalysts listen and imagine that if you hear her lament her mother that would be enough. She praised the woman who did more than just listen."

Dolto has influenced the way babies are treated in some French hospitals where helpers assist mothers who are struggling and try to reassure the baby by constant care.

Body image and multiple personality disorder

Is your body image impacted by personality disorder? Psychologists have been grappling with this intriguing issue since the early 19th century. The question of multiple personality interested some of the best minds of the 19th century – William James, Robert Louis Stevenson, and Pierre Janet. In terms of body image, it raises the question of whether those who have multiple personalities have multiple body images?

In 1995 I attended a conference on multiple personality. Some doctors there were treating patients who claimed to have 200 or so different personalities and many of them reported having different body images. One 57-year-old overweight woman said that some of her alters were six years old with very young, agile bodies. Others were in their teens with raging hormonal bodies. She said "Since there are tons of alters in my system, each of them has their own body image. These include male and female."

She added "Even after almost three decades of intensive psychotherapy, I feel disconnected with my body. My form is getting older and not doing very well. Also, my legs are swollen, and I have begun to feel the pain of arthritis. My wheelchair limits my movements, but I often forget that I am not able to always do the things a walking person can do."

The many tests of body image however have little to say about how multiple personalities affect body image.

Theories and Tests of Body Image satisfaction

First, The Body Uneasiness Test (BUT) of 2005, scale developed by Cuzzolaro, Vetrone, Marano, and Garfinkel (not to be confused with the BUTT test, where you ask your friends to judge your butt, as Tom Hanks asks his friend in *Sleepless in Seattle*). The BUT is a 71-item self-report questionnaire. Part A measures weight phobia, body image concerns, how often you monitor yourself, as well as how estranged you feel towards your own body; Part B looks at specific worries about particular body parts, like "are my lips not full?".

It is useful to look at some of the questions of the BUT test. These include:

1 I spend a lot of time in front of the mirror
2 I don't trust my appearance: I'm afraid it will change suddenly
3 I like those clothes which hide my body
4 When I undress, I avoid looking at myself
5 I think my life would change significantly if I could
6 correct some of my aesthetic defects
7 The thought of some defects of my body torments me so much that it prevents me being with others
8 I'm terrified of putting on weight
9 I make detailed comparisons between my appearance and that of others.
10 If I begin to look at myself, I find it difficult to stop
11 I would do anything to change some parts of my body
12 I stay at home and avoid others seeing me

13 I am ashamed of the physical needs of my body
14 I feel I am laughed at because of my appearance
15 The thought of some defects of my body torments me so much that it prevents me studying or working
16 I look in the mirror for an image of myself which satisfies me and I continue to search until I am sure I have found it

The test also asks questions about the shape of one's head and the shape of one's face, skin, hair, nose, lips, mouth, teeth, ears, chin, neck, shoulders, arms hands, knees, genitals, buttocks, and feet and whether you smell, sweat. or blush.

The discrepancy between what you see yourself as and your ideal body image is often used as a measure of body dissatisfaction. Perceiving one's body to be larger than one wants may make one feel dissatisfied and depressed, making one eat less, perhaps dangerously so. There are personality differences too. Individuals who are more concerned with the way they look have more negative thoughts and emotions. Psychologists speak of body-image psychological flexibility. You have that flexibility if you can experience unpleasant thoughts and emotions about your body size in a detached way, without trying to control how these thoughts and emotions are experienced and how much control they exert over what and how much you eat. Any self-report measure is subjective and carries risks. Do you answer truthfully, or do you choose thinner ideal figures, as you assume that is more socially acceptable? Or conform to what you think is normal?

Then there is the question of how much individuals can accurately introspect and be aware of their own beliefs and attitudes. To get round that researchers use so-called implicit measures, procedures based on how long and how accurately people respond under time-pressure. These are supposed to assess automatic, immediate attitudes and beliefs. Subjects do not have time to deliberately evaluate their preference and produce judgments they think will make them look good.

One useful measure for the assessment of actual-ideal discrepancy is the Implicit Relational Assessment Procedure (IRAP). This assumes subjects will respond faster to answers that are consistent with their experiences. Consider an overweight teenager who has been exposed throughout her life to criticism by relatives and peers, who has been repeatedly told that she should lose weight to look better and be healthier. Like millions, she has seen slim models representing beauty and success. This person is likely to be faster in denying than affirming that she wants to be fat, in other words, showing an implicit desire for thinness.

Heider et al. in their article on *Implicit beliefs about ideal body image predict body image dissatisfaction* (2015) examined actual and ideal implicit body image in two groups of Belgian female college students with extreme (high vs. low) self-reported scores in body dissatisfaction. Subjects did two different IRAP tasks. In the first one, they were shown combinations of the phrases "I am" and "I am not" with words like slim, chubby, etc.

On half the trials, participants were asked to respond, as fast as possible, as if they were thin. So, they were expected to select "True" for stimulus combinations such as "I am slim" and "I am not chubby," and "False" for combinations such as "I am chubby" and "I am not slim." On the other half, they were asked to respond as if they were fat (i.e., by selecting "True" for "I am chubby" and "I am not slim," and "False" for combinations such as "I am slim" and "I am not chubby"). The second IRAP task (ideal body image) was very similar, but the phrases "I want to be" and "I don't want to be" were used instead. Participants were asked to respond as if they wanted to be thin on half of the trials, and as if they wanted to be fat on the other half. For each task, a score was calculated based on the difference in how long it took for subjects to respond. Heider and colleagues found that participants with low levels of body dissatisfaction endorsed the implicit belief that they are thin (and not fat) more strongly than those with high body dissatisfaction. Conversely, they found the latter to show a stronger implicit desire to be thin (and not fat) than the former.

None of these studies found implicit anti-fat attitudes. Some found subjects preferred pictures of thin models over pictures of overweight models; that was entirely attributable to pro-thin attitudes and not to anti-fat ones. Participants in Maroto-Expósito et al.'s (2015) assessment of implicit anti-fat and pro-slim attitudes in young women showed similar positive attitudes both to pictures of underweight and pictures of overweight models. This pattern of results was replicated in a later study from the same research group, but only for participants with very low levels of body dissatisfaction. Participants with high levels of body dissatisfaction preferred underweight model pictures. In sum, previous IRAP research suggests that while positive implicit attitudes to thinness seem widespread, attitudes to fatness vary from neutral to positive, depending on individual differences. The evidence suggests that implicit attitudes to fatness play a significant role in the prediction of different body-image outcomes such as body-image psychological inflexibility, body dissatisfaction, and eating disorders.

Psychiatrists also speak of depersonalisation which means you are detached from a sense of who you are. Some 2 per cent of us suffer from this. Loss of identity can be profoundly uneasy and sometimes patients think they are another person. Depersonalisation is a kind of dissociative disorder. There is a link between depersonalisation symptoms, and derealisation, where you have the feeling of being outside yourself and observing your actions, feelings or thoughts from a distance. Some people talk of out of the body experiences. Derealisation is where you feel the world is unreal. People and things around you may seem "lifeless" or "foggy." You can have depersonalisation or derealisation, or both together.

There is also a link with panic attacks and phobic behaviour, so the fact that Body Dysmorphic Disorder (see more on this in Chapter 6) and Social Phobia seem to belong to the same spectrum is not surprising. The BUT Depersonalisation subscale tries to winkle out the instability of one's self concept with questions like, I don't trust my appearance: I'm afraid it will change suddenly. The research shows links between binge eating, body shame and dissociative phenomena which happen when a person feels they are not one united coherent self.

Body image research is international now and it is worth examining one set of tests to illustrate that. The Multidimensional Body-Self Relations Questionnaire (MBSRQ) has appeared in English, German, Greek, Urdu, and Lithuanian. It is a self-report inventory of how one sees and feels about aspects of body image (Brown, Cash, & Mikulka, 1990; Cash, 2001).

Jankauskinė and Mežienė (2011) prepared a Lithuanian translation which was given to 217 Lithuanians recruited from fitness clubs. Naqvi and Kamal (2017) prepared an Urdu translation which they gave to 350 Pakistani university students. 27 of the 34 MBSRQ-AS items loaded onto four factors (Appearance Evaluation, Appearance Orientation, Body Areas Satisfaction, and Overweight Preoccupation).

A different test is also relevant. The Body Checking Questionnaire assesses how much you check your body and "body focused control strategies" (Reas et al., 2002). Its 23 items include how often you check how your bum looks in the mirror. Results reveal three separate factors: "overall appearance," "specific body parts," and "idiosyncratic checking." The first two are self-explanatory; the third means the personal habits you may have of, for example, making sure you don't have some glup dangling from your nostril or that you have shaved properly if you are a man.

Right after diagnostic assessment, photographs were taken. Then subjects were asked to put on a beige leotard – the image conjures up such possibilities for therapy - and to stand in front of a black background. A female experimenter took pictures from the front, side, and back, excluding the head.

Each of the three views were zoomed and blurred, so in total 24 zoom levels were possible. The detail is awesome but since the figures were deliberately headless also strange.

More work is needed to adapt measures of behavioural body image components to explore how patients with eating disorders react when they see their body images. Including social context information and mood (anxiety) or stress induction may be a next step to better understanding of the behavioural component in eating disorders.

Last there is the Body Image Avoidance Questionnaire which is used to measure self-reported body related avoidance behaviour, for example not looking in the mirror (Rosen et al., 1991). The German translation (Legenbauer et al., 2007) revealed three factors "clothing," "social activity," and "eating restraint." Clothing is self-explanatory; social activity refers to how much, or how little, you engage with others and eating restraint discovers whether you try to eat less than you want.

I have shown there are many tests to evaluate different aspects of body image, but what influences how we feel about our bodies? On to the next chapter and the impact of social media.

4 The Effect of Social Media on Body Image

We've looked at how to test attitudes towards body image, but what influences how we feel about our bodies? Social media is an obvious factor. The research shows a tendency to jargon which I have tried to minimise.

Mark Zuckerberg and some friends at Harvard started Facebook in 2004 just for Harvard students and it went public in 2006. It soon became an essential of modern life. And today there is also Instagram, Snapchat, Twitter now renamed X, videoblogging and Tik Tok as well as Snogchat and Intimagram – I've just made up the last two just for fun. Sites which make it easy to upload pictures are very popular but are the pictures real or fake. Faking images does not require months of training – it can be done easily.

About 10 million new photographs are uploaded to Facebook every hour, a fantastic figure which requires some analysis of its consequences. First, social media features the users themselves. Second, people often present an idealised version of themselves uploading only the most attractive images of themselves. Third, social media lets you interact with your peers and comparing your looks with those of your friends may particularly affect how you see your own body image. In the past we compared ourselves with the Jones or Patels next door – did they have better sofas or grow more beautiful roses? Human competitiveness always finds new areas. Social media research is a busy field with much jargon. Annoyingly subjects never look at images but are 'exposed' to them. Still some main conclusions can be teased out which is not always easy as there are some paradoxical results.

Studies on pre-teenage girls and female high school students (Fardouly et al., 2015) have found that Facebook users report higher levels of body dissatisfaction, more 'drive for thinness, internalisation of the thin-ideal, body surveillance (which seems to mean checking

DOI: 10.4324/9781003425878-4

your body), self-objectification, dieting, and appearance comparisons than do non-users. Self-objectification is a process in which a person views themselves as a physical object first and a human being second. As a result, the person can be hypercritical of their body and parts of their body. If you see yourself as not so good looking it can create issues for your mental and emotional well-being.

Posting, viewing, and commenting on images is also associated with greater weight dissatisfaction, drive for thinness, thinking thin is the ideal, and self-objectification among female high school students.

Gone are the days when men did not care how they looked, if that was ever true. Viewing and commenting on Facebook profiles of one's peers were significantly correlated with drive for thinness among both male and female undergraduates. One study shows a positive correlation between overall social media usage and one's sense of body image.

The importance of Facebook for one's social life was associated with objectified body consciousness (i.e., appearance self-worth and body surveillance) and body shame among male and female undergraduates.

Correlational studies, however, cannot answer an important question; are people who spend more time on social media more concerned about their appearance, or are people who are more concerned with their appearance likely to spend more time on social media? Longitudinal and experimental research is needed.

There are relatively few such longitudinal studies, but one study of male and female high school students found that greater social media usage (specifically from Hyves.nl- a social networking site from the Netherlands which competed with Facebook and MySpace) predicted greater body dissatisfaction and more talk about appearance with peers 18 months later. Another study of female university students specifically examined maladaptive Facebook use like seeking negative social evaluations from others and making general social comparisons and found that this type of maladaptive use was associated with increased body dissatisfaction four weeks later. But there were exceptions; a study examining female high school students' use of online games, blogs, Twitter, and Facebook failed to find any association between social media usage and body image concerns at the time or at six-month follow-up.

Fiorvanti (2021) suggests it is not smart to look at images of attractive same sex strangers. Men and women who studied mock social media profiles reported poorer body image and a less positive mood than did those who were exposed to unattractive same-sex others.

Similarly, exposure to "fitspiration" images taken from Instagram led to a more negative mood and body dissatisfaction among female undergraduate students than did looking at appearance-neutral control images. Rather than showing subjects pre-selected images, two other studies asked them to spend time on their own Facebook account and studied the impact on their body image concerns. For example, one study asked female undergraduate students who spend 20 minutes browsing their Facebook account or an appearance-neutral website and found no increase in preoccupation with weight and shape after exposure to either website.

In fact, weight and shape preoccupation decreased after exposure to both websites, but the decrease was greater after exposure to the control website than to Facebook.

Another study had female undergraduate students spend ten minutes browsing either their Facebook account or an appearance-neutral website and found no difference in body dissatisfaction ratings after looking at Facebook or the control website. How much subjects looked at Facebook correlated with worries about face, skin, and hair but only for women who tended to compare appearance more. Unfortunately, subjects looked at these images for 10–20 minutes, which is much less than the two hours people typically spend on Facebook each day. Also, social media does not affect all women equally; Fardouly et al. (2015) found some characteristics like the tendency to compare their appearance more may make women more vulnerable to the effect of social media usage. The evidence is consistent that social media use (particularly Facebook) is associated with body image concerns among young men and women and that this association may strengthen over time.

Research needs more finesse, and it could test which aspects of social media (e.g., comparisons to specific people, viewing specific content) trigger most body image concerns. Eye tracking technology could also be used to help observe and measure eye movements, pupil dilation, where one gazes, and blinking. These all show where you focus your visual attention, what you engage with, and what you ignore. Carter and Luke (2020) offer a good introduction to the subject.

Try not to look at social media so much

Teens and young adults who reduced their social media use by half for just a few weeks saw significant improvement in how they felt about both their weight and their overall appearance compared with peers who maintained consistent levels of social media use, according to research published by the American Psychological Association. Gary Goldfield, PhD, of Children's Hospital of Eastern Ontario Research Institute and his colleagues conducted a pilot study with 38 undergraduate students with elevated levels of anxiety and/or depression. Some participants were asked to limit their social media use to no more than 60 minutes per day, while others were allowed unrestricted access. Subjects who restricted their use liked their overall appearance (but not their weight) better after three weeks.

A study of 220 undergraduate students aged 17–25 (76 per cent female, 23 per cent male, 1 per cent other) and published in *Psychology of Popular Media*, sought to expand the pilot study. To take part, participants had to be regular social media users (at least two hours per day) and show symptoms of depression or anxiety.

For the first week of the experiment, they were all told to use their social media as they normally would. After the first week, half the participants were told to reduce their use to no more than 60 minutes per day. At the start of the experiment, subjects also responded to a series of statements about their overall appearance (e.g., "I'm pretty happy about the way I look") and weight (e.g., "I am satisfied with my weight") on a 5-point scale, with 1 indicating "never" and 5 "always." They filled in a similar questionnaire at the end of the experiment.

For the next three weeks, participants who were told to limit their social media use reduced it by approximately 50 per cent to an average of 78 minutes per day while the control group, averaged 188 minutes. Subjects who reduced their social media use liked their overall appearance and body weight better after the three-week intervention, compared with the control group, who saw no significant change. Gender did not appear to make any difference. The study found that

> "Our brief, four-week intervention using screentime trackers showed that reducing social media use yielded significant improvements in appearance and weight esteem in distressed youth with heavy social media use," said Goldfield. "Reducing social media use is a feasible method of producing a short-term positive effect on body image among a vulnerable population of users and should be evaluated as a potential component in the treatment of body-image-related disturbances."

Self-discipline is a good tactic. You could use your smartphone to time how long you social, as it were.

5 The Effect of Media and Celebrities on Body Image

If you don't want to feel under pressure with how your body looks, it might be preferable (although impractical) to shun all films, TV, video, magazines, and probably billboards, where notions of the 'ideal' body type still dominate.

The use of ultra-skinny models is being scrutinised, and in some cases, models have been banned from the fashion runway. American media are obsessed by the ups and downs of the weight of popular film and television stars and models, though whether this degree of publicity about actresses' (and models') body weights is healthy or harmful remains to be tested. With a few exceptions, notably Rosanne Barr years ago and Queen Latifah more recently, there are few successful, charismatic overweight female media role models.

In *The Devil Wears Prada* Meryl Streep's assistant, played by Emily Blunt, starves herself so she can fit into small fashionable clothes she wants to wear for Paris Fashion Week. Women who see ultrathin characters in films, television and magazines tend to idealise and internalise these models and become dissatisfied with their own bodies: if only I could look like Ms. Pencil Thin. This is "thin internalisation." Women have been led to believe they can thin up – or should that be down – without too much effort. As I have tried for years to shed 5 kilos, I understand both the desire and the frustration.

Recently the singer Ariana Grande has called on fans to be "gentler and less comfortable" about bitching about her and other peoples' bodies. Fans, Grande said were "comparing my current body" to "the unhealthiest version of my body." She admitted, "I was on a lot of antidepressants and drinking on them and eating poorly and at the lowest point of my life when I looked the way you consider me healthy, but that in fact wasn't my healthy. You never know. So be gentle with each other and with yourselves." Stressing that "there are many different kinds of beautiful," Grande suggested fans should

DOI: 10.4324/9781003425878-5

avoid making even "well-intentioned" remarks about how "healthy, unhealthy, big, small, this, that, sexy, non-sexy" people may look. Rebecca Lucy Taylor, another singing star, feels much the same telling *The Observer*, "This is the body I have without killing myself" (*The Observer*, July 15, 2023).

In fact, real women have got heavier – and some like the actor Miriam Margoyles have actually made it on to the cover of *Vogue* as not quite uncovered models. Margoyles glories in her amplitude- see the issue from July 2023.

Signorelli (1997) showed that teen-oriented shows featured advertisements that used beauty in 56 per cent of ads aimed at girls, but just 3 per cent of ads aimed at male viewers. A total of 70 per cent of girls wanted to look like a television character (compared with 40 per cent of boys). Half of those girls did something to change their appearance. The male 3 per cent needs to be looked at again.

Levine and Harrison (2004) have argued also that media exposure leads to dissatisfaction, a drive to be thin, and ultimately to disordered eating. There was a small but positive association between media exposure and impact on body image. The social-comparison theory asserts that we tend to evaluate ourselves through comparisons with other. "Our upward social comparisons could compel us to eat in a disordered fashion and strive to be thin."

Hogan and Strasburger (2008) predicted that people who view more television will reflect media realities, rather than real-world social realities. An ultra-thin woman on television may eat junk food and not exercise which gives unrealistic information about the link between diet and fitness. The relationship was stronger for magazines than for television.

In a study of 10,000 adolescents, Field et al. (2008) found that 8 per cent of girls and 10 per cent of boys reported using substances to enhance muscle mass, appearance, or strength. Boys wanted to bulk up muscle, but girls also reported wanted to lose weight. Both genders were more likely to use substances if influenced by the appearance of models in the media: Field et al. stated "concern with muscle definition and media images may lead young people to use unhealthful products to achieve a more desired physique." The heavily publicised use of anabolic steroids in baseball and other sports venues may influence adolescents, particularly young men. These findings are not trivial. A recent study of 11,000 adolescents, both male and female, found a correlation between wanting to look like media role models and being more likely to use anabolic steroids or unproven protein supplements.

Field et al. (2012) studied a database of 6,770 adolescent girls aged nine to 14 years. Girls wanting to look like characters on television, in movies, or in magazines were twice as likely to be concerned about weight, become constant dieters, or engage in purging behaviours. In a study of 548 middle and high school girls, Field et al found most of them to be dissatisfied with their body shape; 69 per cent believed that their ideal body shape was influenced by magazines or other media images. The more frequently girls read fashion magazines, the higher the likelihood they had been on diets or started an exercise programme to lose weight. The authors concluded that "print media could serve a public health role by refraining from relying on models who are severely underweight and printing more articles on the benefits of physical activity."

Swiatokowki (2016) found an association between reading fashion magazines and symptoms of body dissatisfaction. Young women in a waiting room were given either four fashion or four news magazines before answering a survey. Those who chose a fashion magazine were more dissatisfied with their weight, had guilt associated with eating, and greater fear of getting fat.

Since films feature beautiful men and women it seems surprising that there is only one film called *Perfect Body*. This is a 1997 American film about a young gymnast who develops an eating disorder. In the movie, Andie Bradley wants to take part in the Olympics. When offered the opportunity to train with a top coach she gratefully accepts. At her first session, the coach looks at her, and she feels she has to shed pounds. She starves herself before another gymnast tells her that there are ways around it. "You can eat what you want and not gain a pound." Andie starves and then stuffs herself and then makes herself vomit. Not clever.

She faints twice, both during competitions, and goes to the hospital where a doctor talks to her parents about her health problems. Finally, she joins a support group where she is encouraged to eat as part of her therapy. At the end of the movie, she is seen walking into the school gymnasium and getting back on the balance beam.

The film is especially interesting in the light of the career of the great American gymnast, Simone Biles. Her story is not central to issues of body image, but please forgive the brief digression into mental wellness and sport. Biles withdrew from the 2020 Olympics primarily due to experiencing "the twisties." In these a gymnast loses awareness of where they are in the air while performing twisting elements. She said it was not the first time she had had the twisties on vault or floor, but she had never before experienced them on uneven bars and balance beam. She decided to withdraw after the first rotation of the team final because she felt that she had "simply got so lost [her] safety was at risk as well as a team medal." US gymnast Aleah Finnegan spoke out in support of Biles in 2021: "I cannot imagine the fear of having it happen to you during competition. You have absolutely no control over your body and what it does."

Some commentators accused Biles of being a "quitter" or selfishly depriving another athlete of the chance to compete. But the fact that she decided to prioritise her own mental health was generally praised. She helped kick start discussion about the role of mental health in sports where performance is seen as all that counts. There are no gold medals for staying sane at Olympic Games.

After her time away from competing, in the 2023 World Championships Biles qualified in first place to every event final, except for the uneven bars. She earned her sixth world all-around gold medal and with this became the most successful gymnast of all time at Olympics and World Championships.

Grace and agility are not all she will be remembered for. Biles said she has many techniques to help with her mental wellness, including using the mental health app Cerebral. "Getting the mental health therapy that I need has been really relieving for me, especially being on the road and on tour." Cerebral – Mental Health App is a mobile application designed to help people manage their mental health. It provides users with a range of tools and resources to help them better understand and manage their mental health. The app includes a variety of features such as a mood tracker, a journal, and a library of mental health resources.

Body Image and Race

Back to body image, and a short note on race. Body image and dissatisfaction with one's body vary across ethnic and racial groups in America. Black female adolescents are "more tolerant of adiposity," (body fat) and Asian American college-age adolescents are less so according to Ambady and Rosenthal (1993).

Black young women who are dissatisfied with their body image may be at more risk for unintended pregnancies and sexually transmitted infections. One study revealed that ethnic identity did not mitigate the relationship between depression and body dissatisfaction for females, and a 2006 study suggested little difference in body dissatisfaction among women self-identifying as black, Asian American, or Hispanic.

There has been little research on what makes people enjoy more body satisfaction. Some studies have suggested that good relationships with parents or feeling supported by your social network helps. Presnell et al. (2004) speculated that "theoretically, cognitive factors such as attributional style or perceived control, which have been linked to depression and anxiety, may be associated with body dissatisfaction." We need more research on resilience and protective factors that leads to more positive body image.

There may be two pathways to body dissatisfaction among boys – weight concerns and muscularity concerns. The existing studies do not yield a simplistic "yes" or "no" answer to the question of whether media exposure causes eating disorders.

If boys pump themselves up with steroids, girls try to reduce the calories they consume. A study of almost 7,000 girls (aged 9–14 years) revealed both peer and media influences on purging: girls purging or using laxatives at least monthly to control weight (1 per cent of the sample) cited the importance of thinness to peers and trying to look like models on television, in movies, or in magazines. Girls wanting to look like their media role models had twice the risk of purging monthly. A recent longitudinal study of 2,500 girls from middle through high school revealed that those who were heavy readers of magazines with dieting and weight-loss articles were twice as likely to engage in unhealthy behaviours of purging and laxative use even five years later. Even young girls in elementary and middle school who read fashion magazines were dissatisfied with their bodies and had more eating-disorder symptoms.

A cohort of college women exposed to "thin-ideal television" among 40 prime-time programs was a significant predictor of disordered eating for women of all races. In the same study, women exposed to sports media did not report disordered eating. Girls who read less fashion magazines had fewer eating-disorder symptoms.

To sum up, there is now considerable evidence that the media influence body image and self-dissatisfaction among young girls and women as well as boys and men.

6 Case histories in Eating Disorders, Body Image Disturbance and Body Dysmorphia

We have seen how distortions in our perceptual body image can lead to eating disorders, so I have explored some early history on this topic.

Ancient Egyptians purged themselves every month for three days in succession, believing that human diseases came from food. The Romans had similar thoughts. They would tickle their throats with feathers after each meal to induce vomiting. The vomitoriums at the Coliseum in Rome were so efficiently designed, with 76 spectator entrances at ground level, that the entire venue could fill or empty 50,000 people in just 15 minutes.

I have been unable to find any case histories of ancient Greeks or Romans who had eating disorders. The first recorded histories are of saints which explains the terms used in the past – anorexia mirabilis, holy anorexia, or inedita prodigiosin; all mean a miraculous lack of appetite.

Perhaps the most famous early case took place in Tuscany in the 14th century. Catherine (Caterina) Benincasa was born in Siena in 1347. It is reported that at age six she saw Christ in pontifical vestments above her local Dominican church. One year later she made a vow of perpetual virginity. Meanwhile, her sister fasted hoping that would change her husband's bad attitude. After her sister died, Catherine responded with a massive fast when her parents announced they had arranged a marriage for her. She became a nun after claiming to have a vision of Saint Dominic. She also declared that Jesus came from heaven and gave her a ring as the wedding alliance; thus, she would be eternally married to Christ. Later in life, Saint Catherine told her confessor that she could have conversations with Jesus. For most of her life she just ate vegetables. They did not agree with as she reported stomach pains that did not allow her to eat anything but the holy host. She died when she was thirty-three.

DOI: 10.4324/9781003425878-6

Three centuries later Shutoku Kagawa (1683–1755) described Japanese patients with a "psychic illness" who would not eat regular rice, but only small amounts of food such as chestnuts or tofu for several days, months, or sometimes for more than a year. Kagawa wrote that 'they would always vomit if they were forced to eat' and they showed bradycardia even though they were not extremely emaciated. Kagawa's description of "Fushoku-byo" resembles the clinical picture of anorexia nervosa today. In a later description, Kagawa also describes the case of a nun who avoided eating for a long period – a close resemblance to the Catholic saints and 'miracle maidens' of Western countries described by Rudolph Bell, in his book Holy Anorexia (Bell, 1987).

Parallels between such medieval behaviour and anorexia nervosa now are apparent. In both, a person becomes obsessed: beauty or slimness in present-day society values and austerity or deprivation in medieval society.

There were no such spiritual motives when in 1698 Richard Morton gave two case descriptions of what we could now call anorexia in his *"Phthisiologia: Or, a Treatise of Consumptions,"* a He described these cases as "Nervous Atrophy, or Consumption." The first involved a "Mr Duke's daughter in St Mary Axe." She was eighteen when she "fell into a total suppression of her Monthly Courses from a multitude of Cares and Passions of her Mind, but without any of the symptoms of the Green-Sickness following upon it... her appetite began to abate, and her Digestion to be bad; her Flesh also began to be flaccid and loose, and her looks pale, with other symptoms usual in a Universal Consumption of the Habit of the Body."

The family consulted Dr. Morton only after she had been ill for two years, and then only because she experienced frequent fainting fits. Morton described her as a "Skeleton only clad in skin." He noted her "continual poring upon Books" despite her condition and that she was indifferent to the extreme cold of an unusually severe winter. She refused any treatment and died three months later.

The other patient Morton described as "The Son of the Reverend Minister Steele." He began to fast at the age of 16. Morton attributed his "want of appetite" to "studying too hard" as well as the "passions of his mind." He advised his patient to abandon his books and move to the country, take up riding and drink plenty of milk, whereupon he "recovered his health in great measure."

There seems to have been little writing on the subject till in 1868 Queen Victoria's doctor Sir William Gull described a "peculiar form of disease occurring mostly in young women and characterised by extreme emaciation." He could not work out the cause of the condition could not be determined, but that cases seemed mainly to occur in young women between the ages of sixteen and twenty-three. *The Lancet* (the BMA's in-house journal) published the following extract from Gull's address:

> "At present our diagnosis is mostly one of inference, from our knowledge of the liability of the several organs to particular lesions; thus, we avoid the error of supposing the presence of mesenteric disease in young women emaciated to the last degree through hysteric apepsia, by our knowledge of the latter affection, and by the absence of tubercular disease elsewhere."

Five years later, Gull published his work *Anorexia Nervosa (Apepsia Hysterica, Anorexia Hysterica)*, in which he described three cases: Miss A, Miss B, and Miss K.

Miss A was aged 17 and was greatly emaciated, having lost 33 pounds. She weighed 5 stones 12 pounds (82 pounds). Gull records that she had not had a period for nearly a year, but that otherwise her physical condition was mostly normal, with healthy respiration and heart sounds and pulse; no vomiting nor diarrhoea; clean tongue and normal urine. The pulse was slightly low at between 56 and 60. The condition was that of simple starvation. She refused all animal foods and almost everything else.

Gull prescribed preparations of cinchona, biochloride of mercury, syrup of iodide of iron, syrup of phosphate of iron, citrate of quinine and variations in diet without success. Very occasionally Miss A had voracious appetite for very brief periods, but these were very rare. She was frequently restless and this seemed a "striking expression of the nervous state, for it seemed hardly possible that a body so wasted could undergo the exercise which seemed agreeable."

In Gull's published medical papers, images of Miss A are shown that depict her appearance before and after treatment. Gull notes how old she looked thought she was only 17: As she recovered, she had a much younger look, corresponding indeed to her age, twenty-one; Miss A remained under Gull's observation from January 1866 to March 1868, by which time she seemed to have made a full recovery, having gained in weight from 82 to 128 pounds. The causes of Miss A's condition and explanation for her recovery have not been recorded. **Miss B** was referred to Gull on 8 October 1868, aged 18, by her family who suspected tuberculosis and wanted to take her to the south of Europe for the winter. Her emaciated appearance was more extreme than normally occurs in tubercular cases. He found nothing abnormal, other than a low pulse of 50, but recorded a "peculiar restlessness" that was difficult to control. Her mother said. "She is never tired." Gull was struck by the similarity of the case to that of Miss A.

Miss B was treated by Gull until 1872, by which time a noticeable recovery was underway and eventually complete. Gull admits in his medical papers that the medical treatment probably did not contribute much to the recovery, consisting, as in the former case, of various tonics and a nourishing diet.

Miss K was 14 years old. She was described as a plump, healthy girl until the beginning of 1887, when she began to refuse all food except half cups of tea or coffee in February that year. She was referred to Gull and began to visit him on 20 April 1887; in his notes, he remarks that she persisted in walking through the streets to his house despite being an object of attention to passers-by. He records that she displayed no sign of organic disease; her respiration was 12 to 14; her pulse was 46; and her temperature was 97°F. Her urine was normal. She weighed 4 stone 7 pounds (63 pounds) and her height was 5 feet 4 inches. Miss K told Gull she was "quite well." Gull arranged for a nurse from Guy's to supervise her diet, ordering light food every few hours. After six weeks, she got better and by July 27 her mother reported that her recovery was almost complete, with the nurse by this time no longer being needed.

Miss A, Miss B and Miss K recovered, but Gull noted at least one fatality as a result of anorexia nervosa.

Gull also recommended giving food at intervals varying inversely with the periods of exhaustion and emaciation. He believed that the inclination of the patient should in no way be consulted; and that the tendency of the medical attendant to indulge the patient ("Let her do as she likes. Don't force food."), particularly in the early stages of the condition, was dangerous and should be discouraged. He admitted having previously himself been inclined to indulge patients' wishes.

Gull is deservedly famous for his medical work but also managed to be one of the thousands of late Victorians to be accused of being Jack the Ripper for no good reason.

The question Gull did not consider was why did they not eat. Orbach has suggested that girls who refuse to eat are refusing to be sexual, so they deny themselves food to make themselves as undesirable as possible. The incidence of sexual abuse in eating disorder patients appears significant, according to research from Tice et al.

(1989). Fifty per cent of patients reported a history of sexual abuse while only 28 per cent of a non-anorexic, non-bulimic control population reported similar problems. Several patterns of behaviour seemed related to previous sexual assault. In one, the eating disorder was used to change the body image of the patient and therefore to provide a defence to future abuse. Bulimic women dealt with a projection of repressed anger toward male authority figures. Forty six per cent of the bulimic women seen in the Tice study exhibited some promiscuous behaviour, using sex either as a gauge of their own self-worth or as a means of punishing men. But it is not easy to speak of this. Once disclosure occurs, a dramatic change is usually seen in the patient and treatment becomes more effective. Patients no longer need to deny their sexuality or punish themselves or others.

Bulimia

Another prevalent eating disorder is bulimia which, put simply, is binge eating followed by vomiting. Those who suffer often take laxatives so they do not put on weight. The pioneer Pierre Janet began discussing symptoms of bulimia in the early 1900s in "Obsessions et la Psychasthenie," describing a woman who engaged in compulsive binges in secret.

Vomiting is not good for you. According to the Bulimia Nervosa Fact sheet from the Office on Women's Health (2012) "The forcing of it may result in thickened skin on the knuckles, breakdown of the teeth, and effects on metabolic rate and caloric intake which cause thyroid dysfunction." It is frequently associated with other mental disorders such as depression, anxiety, borderline personality disorder, bipolar disorder, and problems with drugs or alcohol. There is also a higher risk of suicide and self-harm.

Bulimia is more common among those who have a close relative with the condition. The percentage risk that is estimated to be due to genetics is between 30 per cent and 80 per cent. Other risk factors include psychological stress, cultural pressure to attain a certain body type, poor self-esteem, and obesity. Living in a culture that commercialises or glamourises dieting and having parental figures who fixate on weight are also risks.

Taking a person's medical history is difficult, as people are usually secretive about their binge eating and purging habits. It is estimated that 1.5 per cent of girls and 0.5 per cent of boys suffer from it. The disorder became well known because of Princess Diana.

"Bulimia nervosa, the eating disorder Diana developed within a year of becoming Princess of Wales, was not (as Charles's friends have suggested) an illness "which made a marriage go sour," wrote the late Anthony Holden in a 1993 issue of *Vanity Fair*. "It was an illness caused by a sour marriage." Princess Diana also had a troubled childhood which made her want security, something her marriage did not give her.

Come 1995, in an interview with the now disgraced BBC interviewer, Martin Bashir asked her about it point-blank: "It was subsequently reported that you suffered [from] bulimia. Is that true?"

Diana replied that it was true and that she had suffered from bulimia for a number of years. She referred to it as a self-inflicted secret disease which sufferers inflict upon themselves due to low self-esteem and because they don't think they are worthy or valuable. Diana described the full up feeling resulting from binge eating as a temporary feeling of comfort, "like having a pair of arms around you," but noted how this soon turns to disgust at how bloated you are, so you "bring it back up again."

When asked if she had told anyone in the royal family about it, Diana said she hadn't. "You have to know that when you have bulimia you're very ashamed of yourself and you hate yourself – and people think you're wasting food – so you don't discuss it with people," she explained. "The thing about bulimia is your weight always stays the same, whereas with anorexia you visibly shrink. So, you can pretend the whole way through. There's no proof." In the tactful TV drama series, The Crown, we never see Diana binge eating or vomiting.

Princess Diana died on August 31, 1997 in a Mercedes which crashed in the Alma Tunnel in Paris. There have been endless controversies about whether the death was an accident or the result of a conspiracy. My book *Diana Death of a Goddess* argued that there had been a conspiracy, but conspiracies do not necessarily succeed. This is not the place to replay these arguments.

Body Image Disturbance

We've examined Body Image Dissatisfaction in children- a state of mind where you are not happy with the way you look- but Body Image Disturbance goes further and is classified as a disorder.

Vartanian and Porter (2016) began examining the association between childhood maltreatment and body image disturbance as adults. They claim, "To our knowledge, this is the first review of the association between childhood maltreatment and body image disturbances in adults." They argue that the influence of childhood maltreatment is a risk factor for the development of a negative cognitive affective body image and can be compared to other known risk factors such as thin media exposure (i.e., admiring those who are thin) and is seen despite the time gap between maltreatment and body image assessment.

How this happens is not clear but they stress that the family and its tensions play an important role in the development of negative mental and physical health conditions (Bhandari et al., 2011; Brown et al., 2017; Michopoulos et al., 2015). Most trauma therapies do not include work on body image – even though body image seems to be susceptible to therapeutic change (Farrell et al., 2006; Guest et al., 2019; Scheffers et al., 2017). Not surprisingly, body image alterations were identified as some of the residual symptoms of evidence-based, trauma-focused psychotherapies by Larsen et al. (2019). First results on how well body-related therapy adjacent to trauma-focused psychotherapy in women with a history of childhood sexual abuse are promising (Price, 2005). Body-related interventions seem to improve the frequently reported low self-care of traumatised patients (Felitti et al., 1998). Given the influential role of body image on quality of life and psychosocial functioning (Cash et al., 2004a, b; Scheffers et al., 2017), they suggest including work on body image in therapeutic approaches for maltreatment survivors.

A study into body image disturbance and borderline personality disorder by Dyer et al. (2015) suggests that body image disturbances occur in women with borderline personality disorder. Are the disturbances related to eating disorders and childhood sexual abuse, which frequently also occur in such patients?

In 2015 Anne Dyer and her colleagues compared cognitive-affective and behavioural components of body image for 89 female patients with Borderline Personality Disorder (49 with lifetime eating disorders) and 41 healthy participants using the Body Image Avoidance Questionnaire and Multidimensional Body-Self Relations Questionnaire. Within the BPD group, 43 patients reported a history of abuse. Both a history of abuse and a comorbid eating disorder were independently associated with an even more negative body image. Results suggest a disturbance of cognitive-affective and behavioural components of body image in such patients.

To be it is best to be – if not beautiful at least not ugly or different.

Body Dysmorphic Disorder

Body Dysmorphic Disorder is a mental health condition where you spend a lot of time worrying about your appearance. Those affected by this condition worry a lot about how a specific part of their body looks and it affects their daily life. The Body Dysmorphic Disorder Foundation described this disorder as: a mental health condition characterised by excessive preoccupation with perceived flaws in physical appearance. These flaws appear as very minimal or completely unobservable to others but are a source of great distress to the Body Dysmorphia Disorder (BDD) sufferer. People with BDD can be preoccupied with any aspect of their appearance, but the most common focus is facial features, such as eyes, teeth, nose, skin and hair. BDD differs from body image issues seen in other conditions such as eating disorders, which focus primarily on weight and shape.

Individuals with Body Dysmorphic Disorder reported using maladaptive strategies such as worrying and confrontation more often than healthy controls, when they have intrusive and unwanted thoughts. Such individuals often camouflage their appearance, mirror checking or reassurance seeking. They often have recurrent and intrusive thoughts as well as feelings of shame, anxiety and hopelessness. It harms the way they manage socially. Body Dysmorphic Disorder is still an underrecognised condition and only a small percentage of those who suffer get useful psychotherapy.

Muscle Dysmorphia (MD) is a subtype of the disorder. Those who suffer are preoccupied with the idea that their body is not lean and muscular enough. They see themselves as small and weak even if they look normal or indeed muscular. The weed wants to turn into a warrior by exercising endlessly, taking excessive use of dietary supplements, and, sometimes, anabolic-androgenic steroids. They often avoid important social or occupational activities because of these compulsions. MD affects mostly men.

Lambrou et al. (2006) found higher levels of shame in individuals with body dysmorphic disorder compared to healthy controls. Neziroglu et al. (2010) found that the group were more disgusted than healthy subjects when looking at themselves in the mirror. Enter jargon as the group showed a higher baseline 'disgust reactivity'.

Veale and Neziroglu (2010) found that those who had the disorder tended to ruminate, worry, compare themselves to others, try to reassure themselves and even attack themselves to try to control aversive thoughts and images.

Personal experiences show how acute the problems can be. Abby writes on the Brook Advisory Centre website:

> "I've had a very up and down relationship with weight loss over the years and tried a lot of really unhealthy ways of losing weight. These tend to work in the short-term and you do lose weight, but they are not at all healthy or sustainable in the long run. I did this because I suffer with BDD.
>
> For me, BDD means that my perception of myself is warped – so I don't see myself how other people see me. My self-image changes daily, from selfies I take, group photos I see myself in, or just looking at myself in a mirror.
>
> I think this stems from my upbringing in a predominantly white area. I was surrounded by pretty, skinny, blonde, white girls, and that's all I knew from the age of 5. I was so different from them in terms of my skin, my weight, my hair. It didn't make sense and I grew up thinking that I wasn't normal.
>
> I went through a really dark time when I was younger where I wanted to drastically change my skin colour and tried dangerous methods to do this. Looking back, I can see how messed up that was. I think that with everything I went through growing up, I had an image of what I wanted to be and what I looked like in the mirror, nothing added up and it just turned into this massive issue of me not understanding myself or my place within society."

The House of Commons survey

The House of Commons addressed the issue of body image and mental health in 2023 and provided an up-to-date account of current research and the problems it raises.

Their account cited a Mental Health Foundation report in 2019 finding that 31 per cent of teenagers and 35 per cent of adults feel ashamed or depressed because of their body image, To better understand the scale of the issue, the Commons launched a survey on Twitter on April 25, 2022. 1,550 people completed the survey over two weeks. The results were stark:

> 80 per cent of respondents agreed or strongly agreed that their body image had a negative impact on their mental health, with 61 per cent agreeing or strongly agreeing that their body image negatively impacts their physical health.

> 71 per cent of respondents said Yes to the question 'Do your thoughts and feelings about your body image have a negative impact on your quality of life?'

Body image issues can also result in increased health risks for specific groups, from the increased risk of suicide in those suffering from BDD to the total suppression of testosterone and its cardiovascular risks in those taking long-term anabolic steroids. The Government, the Commons asserted, is not doing enough to understand the scale of these risks or to provide the necessary services for those seeking help. The Commons recommended that the Department of Health and Social Care, along with the National Institute for Health Research fund new research to understand what is leading to a rise in body image dissatisfaction across the population including the impact of social media. This is of particular importance in relation to certain groups known to be vulnerable to body image concerns including adolescents, people with disabilities and LGBT people.

In July 2021 one in six children aged five to 16 in England were identified as having a probable mental health issue. The House got worrying evidence pointing to rising body dissatisfaction contributing to poorer mental health in young people, particularly but not only girls.

Online content promotes an idealised, often doctored and unrealistic, body image and the link to developing low self-esteem and related mental health conditions. Despite the Online Safety Bill, the House believes further action is needed in terms of both culture and legislation.

We call on the Government work with advertisers to feature a wider variety of body aesthetics, and work with industry and the Advertising Standards Authority to encourage advertisers and influencers not to doctor their images. The Commons urged the Government to introduce legislation that ensures commercial images are labelled with a logo where any is digitally altered.

31 per cent of those who completed the survey said they had accessed, or tried to access, health services for issues relating to body image in the past.

Of these, 64 per cent felt that their experience of accessing services was either negative or strongly negative. Perhaps most worryingly 55 per cent of these respondents felt that they had been stigmatised when they accessed, or tried to access, these services. One of those surveyed described having gone "to the doctor for help. I was dismissed, I was diminished." The House urged Health Education

England, the General Medical Council and the Nursing and Midwifery Council to collaborate with third sector organisations to integrate the most effective existing training and resources into all training programmes in the next two years.

Kim Booker, one of the lived experience witnesses who suffers from BDD, told the Commons of her experience of seeking procedures that ended up in "filthy" rooms and taking only "10 to 15 minutes," comparing the process to "a conveyor belt ... without any questioning at all."

The Commons proposed that the Department of Health ought to bolster the Healthy Child Programme. The Government should introduce annual holistic health and wellbeing assessments for every child and young person. These assessments should monitor a range of physical and mental health markers including, to ensure early detection of potential health risks, with signposting to appropriate services.

The Commons was not convinced that this was a sufficient priority for the Government. With 72 per cent of our survey respondents answering 'No' to the question 'Do you think the topic of body image and its related health impacts is receiving sufficient attention from national policymakers?' and only 8 per cent answering 'Yes,' the public agree.

The House urged the Government to immediately initiate a comprehensive cross-government strategy that brings together, at the very least, the Department of Health and Social Care, the Department for Digital, Culture, Media and Sport, and the Department for Education to tackle the current growing problem of body dissatisfaction and its related health, educational, and social consequences. This strategy should include, but not be limited, to education about self-worth, body positivity, critical thinking, and appraising images, as well as wider health advice such spotting signs and symptoms of eating disorders, anxiety and depression and body dysmorphia, within educational, health and online/media settings.

The Women and Equalities Committee's 2021 report, Changing the Perfect Picture found the most persistent causes of body image dissatisfaction to be:

- § Colourism–discrimination affecting people of colour where lighter-coloured skin is viewed as more desirable.
- § Weight stigma–those with a higher body and lower body weight than the average can be subject to prejudice and discrimination.

- § Exposure to media depicting unrealistic and narrowly defined appearance ideals.
- § Appearance-related bullying and/or sexual harassment.
- § The emphasis on the importance of image/beauty in society.

The Commons heard that certain groups were identified as most vulnerable to suffering from body image dissatisfaction. These included:

- § Adolescents – we received evidence that body dissatisfaction is increasing for both teenage boys and girls, however, the motivations behind this may differ.
- § Underweight and overweight individuals – the latter group owing largely to weight bias.
- § LGBT individuals (particularly gay men and transgender individuals).
- § People with disabilities or living with a visible difference.

The Commons learnt that poor body image develops early, establishes itself in female adolescence and is becoming more common. Girlguiding told the Commons that results from their survey showed that in 2011, 73 per cent of girls aged seven to 21 were happy with how they looked, falling to 70 per cent in 2018. However, this masks some of the differences across the age groups, including a significant decline for the 17–21-year age group (69 per cent were happy with how they looked in 2009 compared to 57 per cent in 2018). In addition, they found that at age seven to 10, 51 per cent of girls say they are "very happy" with how they look. By age 11–16, this has decreased to 16 per cent.

The development of poor body image at a young age for girls aligns with what Kim Booker, said: "I have had issues with my body image from as young as I can remember, since about the age of five. That is the body dysmorphia. It would be as minute as me not liking the arrangement of freckles on my knees or the way that my toes were shaped. At that young age – it was the early 1990s – I was growing up in an environment where it was very much the Disney ideal. It was the princess look. As a child, seeing that and being bombarded with those images, I felt that I needed to fit the template of the big eyes, the small nose, the flowing hair, and the tiny waist. That has grown with me through my teenage years, into adulthood. Men and boys also experience body image dissatisfaction."

The Mental Health Foundation told the Commons that 28 per cent of men aged 18 and above had felt anxious about how their bodies looked while 11 per cent had felt suicidal. As with girls, a pattern of issues developing at an early stage was noted, with a survey by

Credos, an advertising think-tank, in 2016 finding that 10 per cent of secondary school boys have skipped a meal to change how they look.

Changing Faces highlighted that three-quarters of men 'with a visible difference' say that men are under pressure to meet macho male stereotypes and that men do not talk about their appearance, suggesting that existing stigma about body image issues may be masking the true prevalence of issues within boys. Charlie King, said how as a man, his struggles with his sexuality added to the development of body image issues at a young age:

> You start feeling pressures. I started feeling pressures within myself.
>
> Because I had not identified with my sexuality then, I was going above and beyond to try to be something that I was not. There was a lot going on. In that period of my life, there was a lot of focus on my image. I was being very critical, I noticed. I wanted to be like the cool guys.

The Commons also heard evidence describing the unexpected ways that body image issues can develop and take root. Another lived experience witness, James Brittain-McVey, described the insidious process by which body image issues developed and was keen to draw a distinction between some people's perception that vanity drives body image issues and the reality experienced by those suffering from those issues:

> One of the biggest misconceptions in my opinion is people presuming that this was striving for vanity because I absolutely loved myself. That was not what it was. There was a degree of self-destruction in my mind about how I looked. There was also pressure to conform to stereotypes and gender constructs. Before I realised, my whole life was controlled by the chase to look a certain way... Without realising, I still had unanswered demons in my head about my body.
>
> Alex Light, another lived experience witness, was clear in stating that "it is not a vanity issue... and [the attitude] that it is something purely for vanity ...prevents people from getting the help they need.

The Commons recommended that the Department of Health and Social Care, along with the National Institute for Health Research, Commission and fund new research to understand the causal pathways that are leading to a rise in body image dissatisfaction across the population and the impact of social media on body image. This is of particular importance in relation to groups that are known to be particularly affected by body image dissatisfaction: for example, adolescents, people with disabilities and LGBT people.

Dr. Georgina Krebs of University College London summarised the clear relationship:

> It is well established that poor body image is associated with a wide range of mental health difficulties. There have been longitudinal studies showing that body image problems in early adolescence are the strongest predictor of the development of eating disorders, for example.
>
> To put that in numbers, individuals who have high levels of body dissatisfaction are four times more likely to develop an eating disorder. Beyond those body image disorders, we know that poor body image is linked with a variety of other mental health difficulties such as anxiety, depression and suicidality. Looking at the research, individuals with high levels of body dissatisfaction are twice as likely to attempt suicide.

The House received much evidence detailing one of the conditions that can directly develop because of poor body image: BDD.

The Commons found that BDD was previously thought to be rare, but recent studies show that about 2 per cent of the general population experience BDD at any one point in time. It is known, however, that the prevalence of BDD is much higher in certain groups. For example, the Mental Health in Young People 2017 survey, commissioned by NHS Digital and conducted by the Office for National Statistics, found that more than one in 20 (5.6 per cent) 17- to 19-year-old girls experience BDD.

The House noted that, among young people attending mental health services for BDD, one in three are out of school because of their appearance concerns. It is also common for young people with BDD to completely withdraw from social activities because of their appearance concerns, and even become housebound. This echoes the experience of Kim Booker who described how it felt to live with BDD:

Rather than see myself as a whole, I see myself as fractured pieces. I home in and zoom in on certain parts of myself and heavily criticise parts that I see as flaws. When I have really bad flare-ups, it can take up about 80 per cent of my mind capacity. It is all I can think about. For instance, when I want to change certain features of my face, I am constantly thinking about how I am going to change it. I feel ugly. I do not like people looking at certain sides of my face. Sometimes I do not want to leave the house.

It is in the category of OCD; it is a compulsive disorder. We ruminate and cannot stop seeing the flaws, even though other people probably cannot see them.

Most worryingly, the BDD Foundation estimated that 85 per cent of individuals with BDD do not get an accurate diagnosis, due both to sufferers being reluctant to seek help and to healthcare professionals lacking adequate knowledge about the condition. We are concerned at the lack of resources being directed toward the treatment of those suffering, many unknowingly, with BDD.

The Commons concluded "We urge the Department to ensure more is done to make the diagnosis and treatment of Body Dysmorphic Disorder (BDD) a priority. From a diagnostic perspective, we recommend that Health Education England update the IAPT (Improving Access to Psychological Therapies) and EMHP (Educational Mental Health Practitioner) curricula to make training in BDD compulsory for all mental health practitioners. As well as improved diagnosis rates, suitable care for those living with BDD must be available. We recommend that BDD specialist practitioners are eventually embedded into the multidisciplinary teams in every new community model for adults severely affected by mental illness."

Dancers

Some professional groups have to be especially aware of their body image. Ravaldi (2003), the author of one of the few relevant studies, surveyed 113 female non-elite ballet dancers, 54 female gymnasium users, 44 male non-competitive body builders, 105 female controls and 30 male controls using the Body Uneasiness Test, the State-Trait Anxiety Inventory, the Beck Depression Inventory, and the Eating Disorder Examination 12th edition (EDE-12).

The ballet dancers might not be Royal Ballet standard but reported the highest prevalence of eating disorders (anorexia nervosa 1.8 per cent; bulimia nervosa 2.7 per cent; eating disorders not otherwise specified 22.1 per cent), followed by gymnasium users (anorexia nervosa 2.6 per cent). All are signs of a high degree of body uneasiness and inappropriate eating attitudes and behaviours.

What can help

Most patients with body dysmorphic disorder look for costly surgical, dermatologic, and dental treatments. But surgery often makes the symptoms worse (Sarwer & Crerand, 2008). Concerns about this led to adverts for cosmetic surgery that target under-18s being banned from May 25, 2022.

The new rules from the Committee of Advertising Practice cover both surgical and non-surgical interventions such as breast augmentation, abdominoplasty, blepharoplasty, injectable fillers such as Botox, chemical peels, and non-ablative laser treatments.

Companies will no longer be able to advertise such procedures around television programmes likely to appeal particularly to under-18s.

Several studies have found Cognitive Behaviour Therapy can reduce Body disorder severity and related symptoms such as depression (McKay, 1999; McKay et al., 1997; Rosen et al., 1991; Veale et al., 1996; Wilhelm et al., 1999; Wilhelm et al., 2011; Wilhelm et al., 2014).

Individuals with Body Dysmorphic Disorder often overestimate the importance of how we think we look to ourselves and others. So, one idea is that patients should focus on minor aspects of appearance as opposed to seeing the big picture. Clinical observations and neuropsychological and neuroimaging findings support this view. (Feusner et al., 2001; Feusner et al., 2010).

Clinicians should ask about thoughts, behaviours, and impairment as symptoms are often undetected in clinical settings (e.g., Grant et al., 2002), owing to embarrassment and shame. The way a patient looks can offer clues such scarring due to skin picking and wearing clothes that camouflage, ideas or delusions of reference, panic attacks (e.g., when looking into the mirror), depression, social anxiety, substance abuse, and suicidal ideation as well as being housebound. In particular, a doctor needs to investigate eating disorders, obsessive compulsive disorder, depression, and social phobia.

Treatment should introduce patients to common cognitive errors such as "all-or-nothing thinking" (e.g., "This scar makes me completely disgusting" or "mindreading" as "I know my girlfriend wishes I had better skin." Patients are encouraged to monitor their thoughts and identify cognitive errors (e.g., "Why am I so nervous about riding the subway?" "I know others are staring at my nose and thinking how ugly it looks." Only then doctor and patient can start to evaluate thoughts with the patient (e.g., Rosen et al., 1991; Veale et al., 1996; Wilhelm et al. 2013). While it is often helpful to evaluate the validity of a maladaptive thought (e.g., "What is the evidence others are noticing or judging my nose?"), it can also be beneficial to examine its usefulness (e.g., "Is it really helpful for me to think that I can only be happy if my nose were straight?"; Wilhelm et al., 2013), particularly discuss the issue of poor insight.

Common core beliefs include I'm unlovable" or "I'm inadequate" (Veale et al., 1996). They can also be identified using the downward arrow technique, which involves the therapist asking repeatedly about the worst consequences of a patient's beliefs (e.g., for the thought "People will think that my nose is huge and crooked," the therapist would ask: "What would it mean if people noticed your nose was big/crooked?") until the core belief is reached (e.g., "If people noticed that my nose was big/crooked, they wouldn't like me and this would mean that I am unlovable."; Wilhelm et al., 2013).

The patient should describe her or his body while standing two to three feet from a mirror. Instead of judgmental language (e.g., "My nose is huge and crooked."), patients learn to describe themselves more objectively ("There is a small bump on the bridge of my nose"). The therapist encourages the patient to refrain from rituals, such as focussing on disliked areas or touching certain body parts. Patients are encouraged to practice attending to other things in the environment (e.g., the content of the conversation, what his meal tastes like) as opposed to his own or others' appearance (Wilhelm et al., 2013).

Specific strategies may be needed to counter some symptoms like skin picking/hair pulling. Patients with significant shape/weight concern, including those suffering from muscle dysmorphia often benefit from psychoeducation and cognitive-behavioural strategies. If patients think surgery will help it is useful to explore the pros and cons of going under the knife. (Wilhelm et al., 2013). Depression is common in patients and may interfere with treatment (Gunstad & Phillips, 2003).

7 Are You Fit to Exercise?

Fitness has always been tied up with body image, and I'd like to begin this chapter on dieting, fitness, and the beauty industry by introducing the Swedish doctor who first made the exercise machines available to the general public.

Dr. Jonas Zander popularised the connections between working out and well-being. He was always on the lookout for opportunities to turn the natural into the mechanical. He could not see a horse without thinking there was no need for a flesh and blood steed. A mechanical horse would do as well, and you wouldn't have to muck out the stables.

Zander was born in Stockholm in 1835. He was weak and sickly as a child. Eager to improve his physique, he studied the ideas of an amateur gymnast, Pehr Henrik Ling, who devised a system of springs and weights that he attached to pulleys. The punter had to strap him or herself in and pull. At medical school in the early 1860s, Zander learned about the mechanics of muscles and joints, and realised the power of resistance to build muscles.

Zander became famous. He took his machines across the Atlantic. An 1895 article in *The New York Times* described the 100 or so pieces of apparatus available at Zander's 59th Street outpost. *The New York Times* noted:

> Every part of the body has its own particular device, even the fingers, one machine being especially arranged for the counteraction of writers' cramps by exercising the stiffened joints.

The age of the Zander Institute was also the age of the electric corset, the Kodak camera and the car. His machines coincided, as well, with the rise of the white-collar worker – and of the kind of sedentary professional lifestyle we now are told to avoid.

DOI: 10.4324/9781003425878-7

The treadmill, which is now the most popular piece of cardiovascular exercise equipment, was first introduced in 1875, and for years it was used in prisons like Brixton in south London. Prisoners pressed down with their feet on steps embedded in the wheel, which moved it, presenting them with the next step. Picture it like the sport of log-rolling, only the log-like wheel was fixed in place. The Brixton treadmill was hooked up to subterranean machinery that ground corn. It wasn't fun.

This treadmill could busy as many as 24 prisoners, standing side-by-side along the wheel.

In a poem about his incarceration, Oscar Wilde wrote: "We banged the tins, and bawled the hymns, /And sweated on the mill: /But in the heart of every man /Terror was lying still."

When America joined The Great War in 1917, the lack of Yankee fitness was worrying. The military tested millions of men. Despite all the exercise machines available volunteers often weren't fit at all. One third of the 3 million Americans tested were too physically weak to be allowed to carry a gun.

Then in 1952, at the University of Washington in Seattle, Robert A. Bruce began using treadmills for human stress tests. He turned them into a consumer exercise device that would allow someone to run or jog naturally while staying in place. In the 1960s the American mechanical engineer William Staub created a home fitness machine called the PaceMaster 600. He began manufacturing home treadmills in New Jersey. (He used it often himself, right up until the months before his death at the age of 96.)

By the 1960s treadmills were common in homes and gyms. Elliptical machines, which are similar in function to treadmills but place less stress on the lower body, were first produced in the mid-1990s and have rivalled treadmills in popularity ever since.

Suffer to get in shape – the mystery of masochism

We are willing to suffer and suffer to improve to look better. More than four million people have taken part in the endurance event Tough Mudder since it was founded in 2010; 20,000 of them have Tough Mudder tattoos. CrossFit has more than four-and-a-half million devotees – more than the population of Wales.

Social media has made obstacle course races popular. Speaking of his experience of competing in Tough Guy, the film's director, Keneally, says:

> "I felt like quitting with every step. It was, at that point, the single most miserable experience of my life." When he crossed the

> finish line, he felt nothing but cold and exhaustion. "Then, a couple of hours later, when I finally thawed out, I felt like a goddam king – like an entirely different person. In retrospect, Tough Guy was one of the most transformative experiences of my life."

The market for masochism is booming. Shortly before the first of his four consecutive CrossFit Games wins in 2011, Rich Froning wrote a line about Jesus's crucifixion on his trainers, taken from the Bible. "If I ever got tired and looked down at my shoe," he explained, "I [would think], 'This is nothing compared to what He went through for us.'" Many footballers and other athletes cross themselves as they take the field though I have yet to see a cricketer do so.

Where there's pain, there can be gain. You stress your body, so it adapts to handle more stress. But there are nicer ways to tone up in air-conditioned, central-heated gyms, which could suggest that it is pain itself some people want.

The question is: why should we seek suffering? Pain can be meditative, meaningful and even pleasurable. In our increasingly cosseted and secular society, pain could ironically be the opium of the masses. The Nobel Prize-winning psychologist the late Daniel Kahneman called this the "satisfaction treadmill": you have to keep running just to feel OK. You may see pain and pleasure as opposites, but the brain doesn't draw such a neat distinction. Both trigger the release of neurotransmitters called opioids and dopamine. They make you "like" a pleasurable experience and "want" more of it. But opioids are also painkillers and stay in your brain for a while after you stop doing whatever was painful enough for them to be released.

William Bridel of the University of Calgary, Canada has interviewed amateur Ironmen to try to understand why anyone would choose something so gruelling as a "leisure" activity. "A few saw pushing their bodies to the limit as pleasurable. "But I'd say the majority positioned it as a way to prove they could tolerate the pain they'd face." Not so much masochism, then, as self-mastery.

Another principle is "hedonic reversal" which occurs when you trigger and override your body's threat response, safe in the knowledge that there is no real danger: by watching a thriller, say, or scaling the final wall in an adventure race. Whether you see these as a challenge or a threat determines whether your pain becomes a positive. The greater your capacity for pain, the less threatening it becomes.

Exposure makes pain more bearable according to experiments at the University of Nebraska-Lincoln. Rats got repeated electric shocks.

They quickly improved their ability to release adrenalin and noradrenaline, readying their body for fight or flight. However, those that received large shocks seemingly at random soon stopped trying to avoid zaps; their adrenalin was too depleted. Meanwhile, those that were exposed to milder shocks and allowed to recover in between – pain training, in other words – fought harder to escape.

Exposure to pain – particularly that you can control – makes you more resilient, physically and also mentally, because the same areas of the brain are involved in both.

Wellness and weight loss

The novelist and former magazine editor Jessica Knoll described her devotion to cleanses, intermittent fasting and elimination diets to make herself look attractive.

> "At its core, 'wellness' is about weight loss," she writes, continuing, "The diet industry is a virus, and viruses are smart. It has survived all these decades by adapting, but it's as dangerous as ever. In 2019, dieting presents itself as wellness and clean eating, duping modern feminists to participate under the guise of health."

Jules Miller, founder and CEO of The Nue Co. has commented:

> The wellness industry sells an unreachable utopia, dictated by rules and restrictions which in turn detaches you from the only real truth, how your body feels in the here and now. Health is about going back to the small, intuitive things in life. Without having to follow a complex set of rules dictated by an "expert."

Four industries benefit from this search for wellness. Somewhere between 7 and 14 million people in the U.K. are said to go the gym.

Endless diets are advertised. Celery yourself to perfection. Third is the vogue for cosmetic surgery. In the United States people spent over $14 billion on procedures. Fourth, there are health farms which *The Times* reviewed in 2023. Just one review shows what they flaunt and flog:

> **Armathwaite Hall, Lake District**
>
> "Set within 400 acres of woodlands and with restful views over Lake Bassenthwaite, the spa at this unpretentious Victorian mansion has employed a forest-bathing specialist – yes, really – to devise retreats that centre on a meditative journey through its

> dappled woods to gain an appreciation of how nature can be a metaphor for change. The brave can try tree-climbing, courtesy of the majestic oaks and twisting groves of rhododendron in the parklands, the hardy can opt for lake swimming."

And if you prefer something quirkier, there are also mindful walks with alpacas. Hugging an alpaca burns calories.

Another personal note

A girlfriend many years ago took me to such a place. I was obliged to exist on under 500 calories a day. I became irritable. It's a miracle our relationship survived for a few more months but once we were out of the starve yourself setting, we did go to some nice restaurants.

Weight loss drugs

Big Pharma also offers dieting help at a price. In The New Yorker Jia Tolentino reported on Ozempic, named perhaps to sound a little like Olympic. Ozempic was developed to combat diabetes but now combats calories. Semaglutide, which sounds less snazzy than Ozempic, ensures the pancreas release enough insulin when the blood glucose level is high. As a result, you feel fuller, so you eat less. It is not without side effects though. Yes, you lose weight but it can show most on the face which has its disadvantages. The skin of the face loses its ability to retract after rapid weight loss due to reduced levels of elastin and collagen. As a result, people taking Ozempic may report – increased signs of aging, such as more lines and wrinkles, loss of fat, which can lead the skin to become loose and sagging. Also, a hollowed-out appearance. Yes, you look like a ghost or someone who has just seen Dracula. You suffer unghostly symptoms though like constipation and diarrhoea. If you have diabetic eye disease and are using insulin, then Ozempic may affect your vision, and this may require treatment.

"The GLP-1 family of medications are highly effective as a treatment for obesity — and therefore should be used as such, regardless of whether patients have comorbid type 2 diabetes," according to Dr. Andrew H. Hogan, professor with the Metabolic Immunology Research Group at Maynooth University, Ireland. "So far, they've been shown to be more effective than other medications we have. So, until something better comes along, that seems to be the best we have medication-wise," he said.

While semaglutide does help people lose weight, they often do not maintain that weight loss after treatment ends. You might imagine that would discourage its use, but it does not seem to do so. We remain obsessed with losing weight. Ozempic is now recommended for the treatment of addiction.

8 Tattoos and Body Piercings

A London tube 2023; there are many people with visible tattoos. When you tattoo yourself or pierce your body, you are choosing to alter your body image. Why do people decide to do that? It is sometimes done just for the hell of it, it seems. There are also T shirts with blazons which usually trumpet you're the tops like 'I am greatness' and 'I am just like you only smarter and better looking'. Subtle. Tattoos are arguably more interesting.

In a supermarket I queue behind a man whose neck is totally tattooed. In April 2024 ITV covered the case of a 79-year-old woman who had herself tattooed with Snoopy. I also met Celine in a bar. She is a lawyer and when I asked her why she had tattoos she rejected any deep explanations. 'I just felt like it.' She was with her sister who was tattoo free. Norwich has a tattoo parlour for every 2,600 people.

The practice of tattoos is very old. The oldest discovery of tattooed human skin to date is found on the body of Ötzi the Iceman, dating to between 3370 and 3100 BCE. He had 61 tattoos. Other tattooed mummies have been recovered from at least 49 archaeological sites, in Greenland, Alaska, Siberia, Mongolia, western China, Egypt, Sudan, the Philippines, and the Andes. These include Amunet, Priestess of the Goddess Hathor from ancient Egypt (c. 2134–1991 BCE).

The ancient Greeks and Romans used tattooing to mark slaves, criminals, and prisoners of war. According to Robert Graves in his The Greek Myths, tattooing was common among certain religious groups in the ancient Mediterranean world, which may have contributed to the prohibition of tattooing in Leviticus. In 316 CE Emperor Constantine I made it illegal to tattoo the face of slaves as punishment.

Fast forward to the 16th century. When Antonio Pigafetta of the Magellan expedition (c. 1521) first met the Visayans of the islands, he described them as "painted all over." The original Spanish name for the

DOI: 10.4324/9781003425878-8

Visayans, "Los Pintados" ("The Painted Ones") was a reference to their tattoos.

> "Besides the exterior clothing and dress, some of these nations wore another inside dress, which could not be removed after it was once put on. These are the tattoos of the body so greatly practiced among Visayans, whom we call Pintados for that reason. For it was custom among them, and was a mark of nobility and bravery, to tattoo the whole body from top to toe when they were of an age and strength sufficient to endure the tortures of the tattooing which was done (after being carefully designed by the artists, and in accordance with the proportion of the parts of the body and the sex) with instruments like brushes or small twigs, with very fine points of bamboo." "The body was pricked and marked with them until blood was drawn. Upon that a black powder or soot made from pitch, which never faded, was put on.
>
> The whole body was not tattooed at one time, but it was done gradually.
>
> In olden times no tattooing was begun until some brave deed had been performed; and after that, for each one of the parts of the body which was tattooed some new deed had to be performed. The men tattooed even their chins and about the eyes so that they appeared to be masked.
>
> Children were not tattooed, and the women only one hand and part of the other. The Ilocanos in this island of Manila also tattooed themselves but not to the same extent as the Visayans."
>
> Francisco Colins, Labor Evangelica (1663)

Pilgrims to the Holy Lands throughout the 17th century were tattooed with the Jerusalem cross to commemorate their voyages. William Dampier was an explorer and pirate who sailed the Pacific in the early 18th century. He rescued Alexander Selkirk (the model for Robinson Crusoe) and landed in Northern Australia before Cook. He brought Jeoly, a South Sea islander, with him to London, intending to recoup the money he lost while at sea by displaying Jeoly to curious crowds. Dampier renamed him "Prince Giolo" and claimed he was the son and heir of the "King of Gilolo." He also claimed that Jeoly's tattoos were created from an "herbal paint" that rendered him invulnerable to snake venom, and that the tattooing process was done naked in a room of venomous snakes. Dampier first toured around with Jeoly, showing his tattoos to large crowds and eventually, Dampier sold Jeoly to the Blue Boar Inn in Fleet Street.

Cook's expedition

Between 1766 and 1779 Captain James Cook made three voyages to the South Pacific. In Tahiti in July 1769, he first noted his observations about the way the natives marked their bodies and that is the first recorded use of the word tattoo to refer to the permanent marking of the skin. In the ship's logbook he recorded: "Both sexes paint their Bodys, Tattow, as it is called in their Language. This is done by inlaying the Colour of Black under their skins, in such a manner as to be indelible." Cook went on to write:

> "This method of Tattowing I shall now describe...As this is a painful operation, especially the Tattowing of their Buttocks, it is performed but once in their Lifetimes."

Cook's Science Officer and Expedition Botanist, Sir Joseph Banks, returned to England with a tattoo. Banks was a highly regarded member of the English aristocracy and had acquired his position with Cook by putting up what was at the time the princely sum of some ten thousand pounds in the expedition. Cook brought back with him a tattooed man called Omai, whom he presented to King George and the English Court.

19th-century Europe

Tattooing spread among the upper classes all over Europe in the 19th century, but particularly in Britain where Harmsworth Magazine in 1898 estimated that as many as one in five members of the gentry were tattooed. They were taking their lead from the royals. When he was a midshipman the future George V was tattooed in Tokyo.

King Frederick IX of Denmark, the King of Romania, Kaiser Wilhelm II, King Alexander of Yugoslavia, and even Tsar Nicholas II of Russia all sported tattoos, many of them elaborate renditions of the Royal Coat of Arms or the Royal Family Crest.

The earliest appearance of tattoos on women were in the circus in the late 19th century. These "Tattooed Ladies" were covered – with the exception of their faces, hands, necks, and other readily visible areas – with various images inked into their skin. To lure the crowd, pioneer women, like Betty Broadbent and Nora Hildebrandt told tales of captivity; they usually claimed to have been taken hostage by Native Americans who tattooed them as a form of torture. However, by the late 1920s the sideshow industry was slowing and by the late 1990s the last tattooed lady was out of business.

In 1969 the House of Lords debated a bill to ban the tattooing of minors, on grounds it had become "trendy" with the young in recent years but was associated with crime. It was noted that 40 per cent of young criminals had tattoos and that marking the skin in this way tended to encourage self-identification with criminal groups. However, two peers – Lord Teynham and the Marquess of Aberdeen and Temair –objected that they had been tattooed as youngsters, with no ill effects. Theodore Roosevelt had the family crest tattooed on his chest.

Since the 1970s tattoos have become part of global and Western fashion, common among both sexes, to all economic classes, and to age groups from the later teen years to middle age. The decoration of blues singer Janis Joplin with a wristlet and a small heart on her left breast has been called a seminal moment in the popular acceptance of tattoos as art. The Canadian Prime Minister Justin Trudeau has a tattoo.

For many young Americans, the tattoo has taken on a decidedly different meaning than for previous generations. The tattoo has "undergone dramatic redefinition" and has shifted from a form of deviance to an acceptable form of expression.

Wearers of tattoos, as members of the counterculture began to flaunt their body art as signs of resistance to the values of the white, heterosexual, middle-class. The clientele changed from sailors, bikers, and gang members to the middle and upper class. There was also a shift in iconography from the badge-like images based on repetitive pre-made designs known as flash to customised full-body tattoo influenced by Polynesian and Japanese tattoo art, known as sleeves, which are categorised under the relatively new and popular avant-garde genre. Tattooers became "Tattoo Artists": men and women with fine art backgrounds began to enter the profession alongside the older, traditional tattooists.

Why do people choose to tattoo their body?

Some inmates of Auschwitz were tattooed using a special metal stamp that gave them a number. They had no choice, just as slaves did not.

Today, being tattooed is very much a matter of choice. One of the most common motivations for getting a tattoo is self-expression. Tattoos can be a way for individuals to showcase their personalities, beliefs, and values. For example, a person may get a tattoo of their favourite quote or symbol that holds personal meaning.

Tattoos can also be a way for individuals to commemorate important people, events, or experiences in their lives. For example, a person may get a tattoo of a loved one's name or portrait to honour their memory.

Tattoos can also be a form of beauty and aesthetics. Some people may get tattoos simply because they find them visually appealing.

When it comes to the impact of tattoos on mental health, expert opinions differ. Lisa Moreno, the founder of InkRevolt.com, emphasises the positive effects of tattoos on mental health, stating that "getting a tattoo can be a transformative experience that empowers people to reclaim their bodies and their identities."

While this may be true for some individuals, it's important to acknowledge that tattoos can also have negative effects on mental health. Therefore, it's essential to make an informed decision about getting a tattoo and to seek support if negative emotions arise.

As Lisa Moreno points out, "there is no one-size-fits-all answer to the question of whether tattoos are good or bad for mental health. It all depends on the individual and their unique circumstances."

If a person experiences regret or negative emotions related to their tattoo, there are several ways to cope. Some people may choose to get their tattoo removed, while others may opt for a cover-up tattoo. It's important for individuals to seek support from friends, family, or mental health professionals if they are struggling with negative emotions related to their tattoos.

Body piercing

Body piercing is the practice of puncturing or cutting a part of body, creating an opening in which jewellery may be worn, or where an implant could be inserted. Piercing implants alter the look of the body and/or skin look (e.g., golden threads installed subdermal, platinum, titanium or medical grade steel). Although there is a lack of scholarly reference, ample evidence exists it has been practiced by men and women since ancient times throughout the world.

The oldest mummified remains ever discovered had earrings, more than 5,000 years ago. Nose piercing is documented as far back as 1500 BCE.

Lip piercings were found in Africa and nipple piercing dates back at least to ancient Rome while genital piercing is described in India round the 4th century CE. Some people pierce for religious or spiritual reasons, while others pierce for self-expression, for aesthetic value, for sexual pleasure, to conform to their culture, or to rebel against it.

As well as the pain of the process piercing carries some risks, including allergic reaction infections, excessive scarring and unanticipated physical injuries. The healing time may vary widely according to placement, from as little as a month for some genital piercings to as much as two full years for the navel.

In the 1960s and 1970s Douglas Malloy's pamphlet Body & Genital Piercing in Brief included such commonly reproduced urban legends as the notion that Prince Albert invented the piercing that shares his name in order to diminish the appearance of his large penis in tight trousers – no wonder Queen Victoria was besotted by him. Some of Malloy's myths were reprinted as fact in subsequently published histories of piercing.

Ear piercing

The oldest earrings found in Ur, the home of Abraham, in a grave dating to 2500 BCE. In Genesis 35:4, Jacob buries the earrings worn by members of his household along with their idols.

In Exodus 32, Aaron makes the golden calf from melted earrings.

Earrings were common in the Eighteenth dynasty of Egypt (1550–1292 BCE), generally taking the form of a dangling, gold hoop. Only nobles had the privilege of wearing gem-studded, golden earrings shaped like asps. The ancient Greeks wore paste pendant earrings shaped like sacred birds or demigods, while the women of ancient Rome wore precious gemstones in their ears.

In Europe, earrings for women fell from fashion generally between the 4th and 16th centuries CE, as styles in clothing and hair tended to obscure the ears, but they gradually came back into vogue in Italy, Spain, England, and France – spreading as well to North America. According to *The Anatomie of Abuses* by Philip Stubbs, earrings were even more common among men of the 16th century than women, while Raphael Holinshed in 1577 confirms the practice among "lusty courtiers" and "gentlemen of courage." The practice of ear piercing among European men spread to the court of Henry III of France and then to England in Elisabeth I's day, where earrings (typically worn in one ear only) were sported by as Robert Carr, 1st Earl of Somerset, Shakespeare and Sir Walter Raleigh. Sailors believed that piercing one ear improved long-distance vision led to the practice among sailors and explorers.

Sailors also pierced their ears in the belief that their earrings could pay for a Christian burial if their bodies washed up on shore.

Nose piercing

Nose piercing also has a long history. c. 1500 BCE, the Vedas refer to Lakshmi's nose piercings but modern practice in India is believed to have spread from the Middle Eastern nomadic tribes by route of the Mughal emperors in the 16th century. It remains customary for Indian Hindu women of childbearing age to wear a nose stud, usually in the left nostril, owing to the nostril's association with the female reproductive organs in Ayurvedic medicine. This is sometimes done the night before the woman marries.

Extreme body piercing: The Vampire

Changes that Maria José Cristerna has made to her body now number an astounding 49 and have earned her a place in the record books. She has done work to her forehead and arms, where she has implants, while she also has a series of piercings and a split tongue.

Her extreme look, where almost 100 per cent of her body is tattooed, has led to her being dubbed a 'real life vampire'.

Robbie Williams Issues Update Over Concerning Posts On 'Self-hatred' And Body Dysmorphia

She said: "The advice I would give is that you have to think about it a lot as it is irreversible. I love the way I look, but you have to understand that there are young people who are very open to tattoos and piercings and everything.

"It's become fashionable, so we might get to a point where it's not what we want anymore, and we might not like it anymore. "So, you have to think about it very hard in order to love it and be able to defend it."

She started modifying her body at the age of 14 and said much had been the most painful to complete. She said: "One of the most painful modifications were the implants in my arms, and also the tattooing of the eyeballs."

The Mirror reported in May 2022 how a body modification addict said children run away in the street after seeing tattooed face, forehead horns, and nose plugs.

The truth is we adorn and mutilate our bodies but there has been little research linking that to body image research. The accent has been on the historical and mythical. So, it seems likely that people choose to tattoo or pierce their bodies for many different reasons. Some may be covering part of their bodies because the real unvarnished body seems inadequate to them, but others may simply be expressing themselves through body art.

9 Facial Disfigurement and Face Transplants

Most research shows that facial disfigurement results in lower self-confidence and a negative self-image that might last throughout life.

Social anxiety, fear of negative social evaluation, and social avoidance are common. People with facial disfigurement worry about meeting new people and find it hard to develop long-term relationships. They often have to cope with teasing, staring, commenting, and asking unsolicited questions about what happened. As a result, people can isolate themselves. Facial disfigurement can also lead to substance abuse and changes in income or occupational status.

Younger patients seem to adapt better especially if it occurs prior to or during puberty. Adults who become disfigured later in life seem to suffer the most and often find it harder to cope with the difference between their "new faces" and "real selves" and are acutely conscious of how others see them. Several studies though have failed to demonstrate a correlation between age, gender, or severity of disfigurement and psychosocial distress.

Perhaps more so than in the general population, in people with facial disfigurement, appearance and self-concept are closely intertwined.

Whether congenital or acquired, facial disfigurement can have profound psychosocial implications, including altered body image, reduced quality of life, and poor self-esteem. The most frequently reported difficulties include negative self-perception and problems in relating to other people because they are confronted with a face that does not look like a face. If you lose a leg, you may well have an artificial leg, different but understandable. The face is individual, unique. While there is not a complete consensus, most research shows that facial disfigurement results in lower self-confidence and a negative self-image that might persist throughout life. Social anxiety, fear of negative social evaluation, and social avoidance are common.

DOI: 10.4324/9781003425878-9

Cleft lip studies have shown that affected children are at greater risk for anxiety, general unhappiness, and self-doubt in interpersonal relationships and that many affected adolescents believe their self-confidence remains affected by their disfigurement. Perhaps most alarmingly, one study showed that the suicide rate among Danish adults with clefts was double that of the unaffected population.

Face transplants are no longer science fiction and can offer new possibilities for those with severe defects. What can be more radical a change to one's body image than having a face transplant? The face is both a biological organ and of identity. In the Harry Potter movies, the Weasley twins are identical but like most identical twins not utterly identical. The face has a unique anatomy and physiology that contribute to its biological functions. Facial skin acts as a barrier, retaining body water and regulating heat. The eyelids keep the eyes moist, the nasal airway conditions and filters air you breathe, and the lips form a tight seal around the mouth so we can eat drink, speak, and kiss. The face has the highest density of free nerve endings in the body.

Face it: you need your face

Treatments for the plastic repair of a broken nose are first mentioned in the c. 1600 BCE Egyptian medical text called the Edwin Smith papyrus:

> "If you examine a man having a dislocation [wenekh] in his mandible [aret] and you find his mouth open and his mouth does not close for him, you then place your finger[s] [? thumb] on the back of the two rami of the mandible inside his mouth, your two claws [groups of fingers] under his chin, you cause them [i.e. the two mandibles] to fall so they lie in their [correct] place! Thou shalt then say, concerning him, one suffering from a dislocation of his two mandibles, an ailment which I will treat. You should then bind it with imru and honey every day until he recovers."

The procedure is so extreme that it merits a number of case histories. Walter Yeo, a sailor injured at the Battle of Jutland, is assumed to have received plastic surgery in 1917.

More recently, nine-year-old Sandeep Kaur's face was ripped off when her hair was caught in a thresher. She arrived at the hospital unconscious with her face in two pieces in a plastic bag. A surgeon managed to reconnect the arteries and replant the skin. Sandeep was left with some muscle damage as well as scarring around the perimeter where the facial skin was sutured back on.

In March 2008 the treatment of 30-year-old Pascal Coler of France, who has neurofibromatosis, ended after he received what his doctors call the world's first successful almost full-face transplant. The operation lasted approximately 20 hours.

On July 18, 2013 the face of a Polish man was successfully given to a Turkish man in a transplant performed by Özkan, at Akdeniz University hospital following a 6.5-hour operation, making it the fifth such operation to take place in the country. It was the 25th face transplant operation in the world. The donor was Andrzej Kucza, a 42-year-old Polish tourist who was declared brain dead following a heart attack while swimming in Turkey. The 27-year-old patient Recep Sert was rushed from Bursa to Antalya for the surgery in late July 2017.

On August 23, 2013 Ömer Özkan and his team at Akdeniz University performed the sixth face transplant surgery in Turkey. Salih Üstün received the scalp, eyelids, jaw and maxilla, nose and the half tongue of 31-year-old Muhittin Turan, who was declared brain dead after a motorcycle accident that took place two days before.

On December 30, 2013 Özkan and his team conducted their fifth and Turkey's seventh face transplant surgery at the hospital of Akdeniz University. The nose, upper lip, upper jaw. and maxilla of brain-dead Ali Emre Küçük, aged 34, were successfully transplanted to 22-year-old Recep Kaya, whose face had been badly deformed in a shotgun accident.

While Kaya was flown from Kırklareli to Antalya via Istanbul in four hours, the donor's organs were transported from Edirne by air ambulance.

Katie: a success story

While a single bullet pierced through Katie's mouth and nasal cavity, exiting her skull between her eyebrows, it miraculously only grazed her brain tissue, but her face was left disfigured.

As Katie herself told the Cleveland Clinic Ethics Committee, during a meeting to ensure she was ready for her face transplant surgery: "I can't go backward. I have to go forward."

"The surgeons were very matter of fact with us. No gloom and doom, but no peaches and cream, either. One of them – an elderly gentleman – said it was the worst case he'd ever seen," Katie's father Robb said.

And then the physician used a phrase Robb had never heard before. "He said, 'Outside of a face transplant, I just don't know.'" "And I'm thinking, 'Face transplant? What is that?'"

Five weeks later, in May 2014, Katie was flown to Cleveland, Ohio, and admitted to Cleveland Clinic. The Clinic have published an account of the case on which this history is based.

On a Sunday morning, the family met Dr. Brian Gastman who would become Katie's primary plastic surgeon. Robb described him as a ball of energy, who came to their meeting armed with a 3D image of Katie's head. Her father said:

> "I'm seeing inside of my child's head. Everything. The wound area, her bone structure. It was fascinating."

Katie's parents have kept a running list of those who have treated their daughter: Nutritionists. Physical therapists. Endocrinologists. Infectious disease specialists. Neurosurgeons. Ophthalmologists. Social workers. Bioethicists. Psychiatrists. Anaesthesiologists. Dentists. Pharmacists. Internal medicine specialists. Vascular surgeons. Dozens and dozens of nurses. And of course, plastic surgeons. Throughout this process, Cleveland Clinic psychiatrist Kathy Coffman, was a key specialist who would talk to her to make sure this is what Katie really wanted.

"Dr. Coffman was speaking about all the risks involved," Katie's mother said. Katie let Coffman finish, and then she said, "I still want to do this, Dr. Coffman." "I want to be able to go out in the world. And not be looked at like this." Katie signed the consent forms for facial transplant surgery in November 2015.

It would be another 18 months before she would be physically and mentally prepared – and the search could then begin for a suitable donor. It would prove to be difficult. Because of Katie was young, the potential donor pool was smaller. And even smaller because the majority of available donors are male.

From the moment of Katie's arrival, the team had the end goal of face transplantation in mind – as facial reconstruction alone would not correct her facial disfigurement or improve her quality of life. Thus, during her preparatory reconstruction surgeries, the surgeons were able to safeguard any potential blood vessels that could be used for the transplant.

"Plastic surgery is about restoring form and function," said Dr. Papay, the Chairman of the Dermatology & Plastic Surgery Institute at Cleveland Clinic. "Function comes before form, and prior to the face transplant, Katie had extremely poor function and form."

At various points during the 31-hour procedure, Drs. Papay and Gastman would leave the surgical suite armed with photos taken during the surgery to discuss next steps and options with Robb and Katie's mother Alesia.

As Dr. Papay explained, "We were well prepared. But we knew our game plan could change in the middle of surgery. And that's what happened. We ended up using more of the donor's face than we originally planned and went to option B about halfway through the surgery," which would increase the risk but improve both the form and function of her face.

Ultimately, with option B, doctors in effect replaced 100 per cent of Katie's facial tissue with the donor's, from mid-scalp all the way down to her jaw and neckline. Further, her upper jaw and the area beneath her orbital floors, as well as two-thirds of her lower jaw, are bone from the donor. One of the trickiest parts of the surgery involved ensuring blood vessels remained functional and sufficiently carried blood throughout her body.

The operations worked. More than 17 surgeries at Cleveland Clinic. Collectively, those procedures have made it possible for Katie to breathe, chew, and swallow more effectively. She's also able to use her face to better express emotions.

A year later Katie has not suffered any signs of rejection, or side effects from being on immunosuppressant drugs, and a series of subsequent operations to fine-tune certain areas (including her tongue to improve speech) have gone as planned.

Beyond the medical triumphs, Dr. Papay is certain Katie would not be on the verge of a new life if not for the constant support of her parents, siblings and extended family. "In addition to the physical trauma that Katie went through is the emotional trauma they all suffered," Dr. Papay stated. "They are about as resilient as you can be, and I am proud of them as much as I'm proud of Katie."

When speaking of face transplants doctors aren't sure what the future holds for these types of surgeries, including the possibility of hand transplants and uterine transplants. To date, most U.S. face transplants have been paid for by the U.S. Department of Defence's Armed Forces Institute of Regenerative Medicine I (AFIRM I) grant programme, which is designed to help improve the treatment of U.S. service members wounded on the battlefield.

"Will third party government and private payers support these patients that are in desperate need of a transplant?" Dr. Papay asked. "The key for (the future) is the source of financial support in these cases."

In a statement that Katie prepared for the media when her face transplant was complete, she spoke of her gratitude to everyone involved. "I am forever grateful for the care this hospital has given me and continues to offer on my journey of recovery and healing," she stated. "And to my donor and her family – words cannot express the appreciation I have for this incredible gift. With a grateful heart, I say thank you to all who have made this possible for me."

Katie's mother believes that in many respects, Katie is just beginning her journey. "I don't know how exactly, but I know Katie will help people. I feel in my heart she will as a mom. I just want Katie to enjoy life and make a difference in society. And I want her to be able to be independent." Rob added, "We have a road to go yet. But we're thankful that we have a road."

Ethics, surgery, and post-operation treatment

There has been much ethical debate surrounding the face transplant operation. The procedure entails submitting otherwise physically healthy people to potentially fatal, lifelong immunosuppressant therapy. So far, four people have died of complications related to the procedure.

Citing the comments of various plastic surgeons and medical professionals from France and Mexico, anthropologist Samuel Taylor-Alexander (2016) suggests that jingoism has played a part because in influencing the decision-making and ethical judgements of the involved parties. His most recent research suggests face transplant surgeons need to do more to ensure that face transplant patients are informed of the risks.

After the procedure, a lifelong regimen of immunosuppressive drugs is necessary to suppress the patient's own immune systems and prevent rejection. This increases the risk of developing life-threatening infections, kidney damage, and cancer. The surgery may result in complications such as infections that could damage the transplanted face and require a second transplant or reconstruction with skin grafts.

I have a brief firsthand account on face transplants. In Israel when I made a film about the medical help Israel offered to Syrian dissidents, I filmed a Syrian nurse who had a full-face transplant. He was amazed to have been so well treated, since he had been led to believe otherwise about Israelis, and he was calm a few weeks after the operation. He vowed to return to Syria to pass on the medical knowledge he had gained.

The after-effects of face transplants

Costa, a Portuguese scientist, who with his team studies the effects of dental surgery, has described how postsurgical facial disfigurement leads to damaged self-concept and takes long to repair. Patients "reorganise perception of self into a once again acceptable unity."

Having to rapidly adapt to new facial features and incorporate them into their self-concept is, patients say, "confusing, frightening, and disorienting" and that even close friends and family members initially struggle with adapting to their new appearance.

Frost et al. describe how patients who have such surgery report temporary depression and loss of self-esteem, but Kiyak et al. report that these alterations in self-esteem and body image stabilise after about two years. In one study by Dorante et al. six patients underwent face transplant. Four had full face transplants, and two partial face transplants of the middle and lower two-thirds of the face. Indirect evaluation showed that expression of happiness significantly improved 1 year after transplant. Expression of happiness was restored to a mean of 43 per cent (range of 14 per cent to 75 per cent) of that of healthy controls after face transplant. The expression of sadness showed a significant change only during the first year after transplant All other emotions showed no significant change after transplant. Nearly all emotions were detectable in long-term direct evaluation of three patients, with expression of happiness restored to a mean of 26 per cent (range of 5 per cent to 59 per cent) of that of healthy controls.

Scientists from Royal Holloway, University of London, the University of Kent and New York University Langone Health investigated the case of a man who underwent the procedure at the NYU Langone Health's Hansjorg Wyss Department of Plastic Surgery. They analysed the patient's recognition of his face, both before and after the face transplant, over a period of 28 months. They examined how the brain responded in a self-face recognition task, the researchers were able to study the brain networks involved in recognising their own face and how they changed over time.

According to the findings, before the operation the patient identified more strongly with what he looked like before his injury. However, after the transplant the patient gradually recognised his new appearance as his own face. The researchers found the medial frontal cortex of the brain – which is involved in various aspects of self-identity – showed similar activation for both their pre-injury and post-transplant faces within 20 months of the operation.

Professor Manos Tsakiris, from the Department of Psychology at Royal Holloway, who led the research, said:

> "While the acquisition of a new face following facial transplantation is a medical fact, the experience of a new identity is an unexplored psychological outcome. Our research set out to answer if recipients of a face transplant would come to recognise their new appearance as their own face. The study's impact on future patient care could be significant as almost all medical conditions result in important changes in the psychological experience of our body."

Nonetheless, over the last decade, various groups have scrutinised and explored the ethical and psychosocial aspects along with how they change self-concept as the face is so vital for self-recognition, self-expression, and interactions with others.

The Royal College of Surgeons of England and the French National Consultative Ethics Committee for Health and Life Sciences [82] did not initially support the procedure. A review of all the literature published between 2005 and 2012 found that the majority of articles cited negative "identity change" and resulting psychological effects as the primary concern. Robertson argues that scepticism about transplants stems partially from the fact that it involves continuation of the deceased donor in a unique way that does not apply to solid organ donors. The symbolic significance of the face can create an emotionally charged and complicated situation for donor families, who might ultimately refuse donation for this reason.

Another crucial aspect of face transplants is ensuring that recipients embrace their new faces. Patients who have a strong preoperative self-concept adapt better to changes and suffer fewer negative psychosocial consequences. Proponents of transplants argue that for these psychologically prepared recipients, the procedure allows them to regain their lost identities. Furthermore, facially disfigured patients report that, in pursuit of regaining their personal identity, they would be more willing to accept the risks of immunosuppression and would tolerate greater risks than patients facing kidney transplants.

Understanding of the long-term psychosocial effects is limited and additional data are needed to better evaluate the risk-benefit ratio of the procedure. There are also potential issues of consent, given that face transplant recipients are so vulnerable – and that "withdrawal" from any trial is essentially impossible. Future research should focus on identifying emotional and psychological factors that correlate with better psychosocial outcomes.

It is also worth noting that face transplants inspired a book 50 years ago. Kōbō Abe wrote *The Face of Another* (1964) about a plastics scientist who loses his face in an accident and proceeds to construct a new face for himself. He then saw the world in a new way and even goes so far as to have a clandestine "affair" with his estranged wife. The novel was made into a film of the same name by Hiroshi Teshigahara in 1966.

I am what I look like now. But I am also what I remember of myself.

10 The Troubled Language of Disability

One of the most remarkable people with disabilities was Arthur Kavanagh who was born in 1829. He called himself a "pink torso." Pink because he wore hunting pink. Despite having only tiny stumps for arms and legs, he could ride and shoot. He had the advantage of being rich, but he did not let his missing limbs stop him becoming a Member of Parliament, travelling to Russia and India and fathering six children.

Franklin Delano Roosevelt, who became President of the United States in 1933, used a special wheelchair he designed himself. Most buildings during his era were not wheelchair accessible; therefore, Roosevelt needed something small, appealing, efficient, and discreet. Ingeniously he used a dining chair and replaced the legs with bicycle-like wheels.

The chair was small and could move around tight corners and narrow hallways. It did not attract much attention, since it was made out of something people were used to seeing in their own homes.

Roosevelt never wanted Americans to get the impression that he was helpless, so it was important to him to at least seem as if he could walk. He devised a method of "walking" in which he used a cane and the arm of his son or advisor for balance. He asked the press not to photograph him walking or being transferred from his car. In that more deferential time, most reporters and photographers complied and if they did not there was trouble. The Secret Service interfered with anyone who tried to snap a photo of the President in a "disabled or weak" state. In TV shows today, being in a wheelchair is no handicap. In both British crime drama series, *Silent Witness* and *Vera*, the police use a woman with disabilities as the lead researcher, both marvels at surfing the internet.

But coping with disabilities is not always easy. In 1990 my small company published a book by Marc Eccleston of the problems he faced after he was injured when jumping and lost the use of his legs.

DOI: 10.4324/9781003425878-10

Marc's book was nominated for the Whitbread Sports Book Prize. He is brave, angry and thoughtful.

Marc wrote:

> "I asked my dad to pick me up when it was dark because I didn't want anyone to see me getting out of the car. When I got to the house it seemed like the whole street was there. I know they meant well but I hated it. I wanted to die."

He said he felt like a circus freak in his wheelchair. However, Marc found a way to restore his sense of self. He played table tennis, became a member of the England wheelchair rugby team and won a silver medal at the Athens Olympics. But he remained bitter though he hoped for some medical advance that would give him back the use of his legs.

Body image in people with physical disability has received little research attention, and I draw on some of the classic research here. Goffman's theory of stigma from 1963 claimed that anomalous attributes result in a negative evaluation and perception of the person with the physical disability. People whose bodies are devalued by society are all too aware of it and may devalue themselves, which may damage their body image. Goffman also proposed that people with more obvious physical differences will be more severely stigmatised and receive more negative feedback.

Wendell (1996) wrote that people with disabilities arouse fear in the able-bodied people, and it is for this reason that they are made 'Other.'

When we make people 'Other', we group them together as the objects of our experience instead of regarding them as subjects with whom we might identify. We see them primarily as symbolic of something else – usually, but not always, something we reject and fear and project onto them. In any case, they must struggle harder than nondisabled people for a self-image that is both realistic and positive which is made more difficult by other people's reactions to them" (Wendell, 1996).

People with disabilities symbolise, among other things, imperfection, failure to control the body, and also everyone else's vulnerability.

Murphy (1995) argued, "the disabled, individually and as a group contravene all the values of youth, virility, activity, and physical beauty that Americans cherish." He drew on his personal experience of living with quadriplegia stating that disabled people are resented by the able-bodied and are seen by them as ugly and repulsive but also they are perceived as subverters of social values and ideals.

Lawrence and Thelen (1991) stated people with physical disabilities feel they do not 'measure up' to the cultural ideal. They may wish for bodies that they cannot have, or they may reject the physical ideals as narrow and oppressive, or they may fluctuate between these points of view (Wendell, 1996). "Emotional tension which is painful and unpleasant may become difficult to reduce or eliminate, leading the individual to feel inadequate, inferior and socially unacceptable (Lawrence & Thelen, 1991).

Mackelprang (1993) observed that atrophied limbs, spasticity, urine bags, and the need for physical assistance could all contribute to low sexual self-image. Rousso (1992) argued that people with cerebral palsy often question how attractive they are as they suffer from uncoordinated, have involuntary movements, and speak in an uneven, unmelodious voice, all the opposite of what is generally thought of as desirable.

It starts young. In a study of 121 able-bodied children on a summer camp, those with a physical disability were less liked and seen as less attractive (Kleck & De Jong, 1983). Cromer et al. (2008) found that adolescents with disabilities had poorer scores on a body and self-image sub-scale than able-bodied adolescents. Another study of over 3,000 adolescents and young adults found that those with chronic conditions scored lower on body image than their able-bodied peers (Wolman, Resnick, Harris, & Blum, 1994). The same was true in a small study of females with spinal cord injury (Kettl et al., 1991). Twenty-seven women completed a questionnaire investigating their perception of their sexuality, body image, and sexual behaviour after their injury. The largest change was the perceived attractiveness of their bodies; the disabled subjects rated their bodies as being only half as attractive after their injury.

Adolescence sees body changes, personality adjustment, and establishment of new personal relationships. The way we experience our bodies is crucial and it is reasonable to admit that physical disability, in some way, interferes in this development. Russo et al. (2012) studied the impact of physical disability in some aspects of the body image, such as self-esteem, body satisfaction, self-concept, and sexuality; the relation between body image, movement and rehabilitee, and the importance of a good psychological adjustment and the professional and social support.

Attitudes to disability have changed to some extent at least, but over half the 14,491 of disabled respondents in the 2021 UK

Disability Survey reported worrying about being insulted or harassed in public places, and a similar proportion reported being mistreated because of their disability.

One person's account is riveting

Ali tells her story on the Disability Horizons website; an online disability lifestyle publication that aims to give disabled people a voice. Ali lost her leg when her wellbeing was "low."

> "I would say when I first lost my leg, I felt a lack of balance. It is a huge adjustment going through trauma so that, yeah. That went on for quite a while […] Like everything is changing. Every aspect of your life is changing. And your disability is going to impact most parts of your life, so it is like everything is uncertain except for maybe like your family or your friends. But even your relationships with your friends do change because unfortunately your ability changes and the things that you do change. So, you have less opportunity to hang out with the people you would normally see."

Ali is quoted on the Disability Horizons web site which reports she felt defiant. "Anything that society told me I couldn't do, I would go on and do it. Any box they put me in, I ran away from. I effectively escaped everything that was part of my identity – and disability was the biggest."

She decided to study for a Master's and then a PhD which was not easy as she found problems with access. She had to get into taxis that did not have ramps, and some, seeing a wheelchair, would not stop to pick her up. They were "For Hire", but not for the disabled.

Ali went to see *The Elephant Man* at the theatre, a play based on a book about Joseph Merrick whose face and body were utterly deformed. And there was a line in it that struck a chord with me: "Sometimes I think my head is so big because it is so full of dreams." I was always told that my head is bigger than my body because it is full of knowledge. Sitting in the theatre and listening to that line made memories I had suppressed come flooding back. I found myself identifying with the idea of the play – seeking acceptance in a superficial world."

Ali said:

> "My body is mine, whatever it looks like. I will now accept and protect it from others, and I won't lie when I am in pain or get

annoyed at it. My body has given me strength that many with 'normal' bodies lack. It's allowed me to discover and see people for who they really are.

Most importantly though, it has provided me with determination to show the world that having a perfect body does not guarantee you the perfect future.

To escape prejudice, I invented an imaginary world in my head, to avoid uncomfortable looks I dreamt of progressing in every path I took and to cope with rejection that often occurred because of my appearance I became immune to hurt. For all these things I am thankful because without it I would not be where I am today."

Multiple Sclerosis (MS) and Body image

There is an increasing amount of research on body image in those who suffer from chronic diseases, but there have been few reports on the experience of body image changes for those with MS. In a study from 2023, supported by the Ministry of Health in Italy, Lo Bueno and colleagues looked at the relationship between body image, disability and mental health in patients with this condition. They found that "the degree of disability was an important risk factor for the development of greater body image-related distress. Physical disability has a negative influence on people's psychological experience, attitudes, and feelings about their own bodies. In MS, the progression of the disease with the consequent loss or alteration of motor functions, sensory and cognitive, seems to cause an increase in psychopathological symptoms related to the possible loss of autonomy and fear of diminishing the reliability of one's body."

The study also found that MS affects one's sense of identity and self-image, but also other spheres of functioning. "In addition, individuals with MS are often plagued by the unpredictability of their disease and have to contend with uncertainty in their life and significant life changes. This can lead to high levels of stress, perceived lack of control, helplessness, depression, and anxiety that can influence their own body image." Men and women with MS also had different concerns. Men were worried about their sexuality, whereas women were worried about gaining weight and becoming less attractive. But in general, for people with MS the concern is that one's own body may no longer be taken for granted but may become instead a disturbing presence. MS leads, therefore, to rethinking the meaning of life, and poor body image can affect physical and psychological health and can influence self-esteem, mood, competence, social functioning, and occupational functioning.

However, some studies differ. A 1978 study found no difference in body esteem between people with and without a visible physical disability (Gruver & Nelson, 1978). Samonds and Cammermeyer (1989) studied the body image of 20 men who had been diagnosed with MS and found that their scores on body satisfaction or dissatisfaction were similar to the scores of able-bodied college-aged men.

Jennie Adams was 19 when she was diagnosed with MS. In an article on the MS Society website, written in July 2017 and entitled 'The invisible symptoms of my MS' she says she sometimes feels walking is like "I'm trying to wade through treacle and looking drunk as a result, to double vision resulting in extreme nausea and hardly being able to stand up or walk in a straight line." She is tired, tired, tired.

She also explains how MS impacts her body. "My body can be suddenly overwhelmed by an intense itching sensation from my head to my toes, leaving me vigorously scratching and rolling around in pain... Due to weakness, my limbs often feel like they have weights strapped to them. When I'm already struggling with fatigue, trying to drag my cumbersome arms and legs around is not helpful. I look incredibly clumsy as I trip over my own heavy feet."

She does not blame people for thinking she is overreacting but "I tell them that either I fight this every day and make sure my life is the best it can be, or I give in. The latter will never happen."

Writer, blogger, and editor Raya Al Jadir, who was awarded the Rosalynn Carter Fellowships for mental health journalism in 2020–21 has written, "It is a natural human instinct to love yourself, but what happens when your body shape or image fails to meet the idea of what is supposed to be 'liked', let alone loved? You become trapped in dual of dislike and love – an internal conflict within you that eventually destroys your self-confidence, leading to possible isolation even when surrounded by many. For some young disabled people, it can be difficult to have good body confidence when you have a physical disability."

Rose wore a back brace which made her feel different and isolated. She attended a mainstream secondary school and she struggled when she would hear the other students laughing or mocking her but resolved not to allow anyone to notice. Raya says:

> "I ignored the bullies and strived to be stronger than their superficial attitude. I studied hard, excelled at most subjects and my

> confidence grew slowly. This confidence reached its peak when these same students wanted my help with their homework and, after a short while, asked to be my friends. I forgave them and accepted their friendship as their taunting was in a way a defensive mechanism that protected their own vulnerability and worries about their appearance.
>
> No one is perfect and we all have things about our bodies that we are not keen on. But over time we have learnt that what you don't like and choose not to 'see', others will ignore too. I ignored comments that reached my ears, stopped looking at mirrors and examining my body and concentrated on things that I chose to see, which inevitable forced others to follow suit."

Raya now feels stronger and feels that what she endured as a child and a teenager has equipped her to deal with such people in adulthood. "They are trapped in a one-dimensional world where being different is a frightening concept. I no longer feel that I am trapped in an unwanted body, but I am trapped in a world with people that are rigid and conventional."

Personal perspectives on body image and disability

Academics Taleporos and McCabe (2002) have spent much of their careers researching body image. In 2002 they wrote a paper on personal perspectives on body image and physical disability, based on a study to investigate the body image concerns of people with physical disabilities. Participants were invited from Monash University, the Muscular Dystrophy Association, wheelchair sporting groups and the first author's peers of disability activists in Melbourne.

The sample was tiny. There were three men and four women. Their disabilities were: two spinal injured quadriplegics; one spinal injured paraplegic; two participants with neuromuscular diseases; one with cerebral palsy and one with a brittle bone disease. The participants were asked about their feelings towards their bodies, how they saw themselves, whether they saw themselves as sexy, or if they felt that their disability made them feel unattractive.

The authors gathered very useful self-reports and I refer to a few of these in some detail. Katie is aged 33, living with her partner. She has severely impaired mobility and uses a motorised wheelchair as a result of spinal muscular atrophy. Katie said she liked some things about her body: "I like the way my hair looks, and I like my fingernails when they're done up and I've polished them, and I like the way

I put on make-up ..." However, she still says she picks fault with every aspect of her body: "There are minor things that I like but basically if I could do a body swap, I'd do one in an instant." However, Katie feels differently about her sexuality which she sees as "such a contradiction: to feel so negatively about your body, and yet so positive about your sexuality." Katie believes that her negative feelings about her body are the result of negative feedback, especially rejection from potential sexual partners.

Sue is a 39-year-old single woman with muscular dystrophy who uses a motorised wheelchair. She considers how her body image has gone through an evolution since her diagnosis: "My body image and sexual image have probably improved as I've become more disabled. Before I was diagnosed, I hardly even thought about my body. When you're 18, every female is young, sexy and every man runs after you. After I was diagnosed, I thought I wouldn't be attractive anymore. I still thought I was sexual, but I didn't think I'd be able to express it anymore. I thought that having muscular dystrophy would put men off and they'd think that I wasn't attractive because I can't walk very well. I was very angry at my body: I felt betrayed. Although I knew I was a sexual being, I thought I wouldn't be seen as that." However, Sue's views have changed as she has grown older: "I used to think that I was deficient as a disabled woman, but as I've matured I've realised that nobody's perfect." She now feels quite happy with her body image and thinks it is pretty healthy – probably even better than some of her able-bodied friends.

For Phoebe, the negative social attitudes towards disability are a challenge. She explains how: "I was waiting for the train one day, and this guy came up to me and said, 'I'm really sorry that you're in that thing', referring to my wheelchair of course, and I said, 'why is that?' He said, 'You know you're really not bad looking, you're really quite pretty, it's such a shame that you're actually in that thing, it's such a turn off'. And I was just blown away, I didn't quite know what to say ..."

The findings from Taleporos and McCabe's study suggests that personal achievement, such as sport, family, career, or education helps, as does focussing on the positive aspects of their body and perceiving the impairment as just one sign of physical imperfection with which we all struggle. Positive feedback from partners and others can also help a person with a disability to achieve a positive body image, even when they do not duplicate the image of beauty that is upheld in our society. Overall, the study provides an insight into the social interaction between able-bodied people and people with physical disabilities from the disabled person's perspective.

Having spotted there was a significant gap in the literature on body image in individuals with physical disabilities, Marios Argyrides and his colleagues (2023) conducted research that set out to explore the relationships between body image, media influences, self-esteem, and situational body image dysphoria in individuals with visible physical disabilities. In their sample of 154 Greek participants and through the use of questionnaires, the findings highlighted the significance of sociocultural influences on body image concerns, as well as the importance of social support in reducing the negative impact of these issues on daily functioning. The study showed that individuals with physical disabilities face appearance-related concerns as a result of sociocultural attitudes which promote an idealised image of beauty featuring socially desirable characteristics, which may be unattainable for individuals without physical disabilities, and even more so for those with physical disabilities (Bailey et al., 2016). Being wise about body image requires you, whether able and disabled, to realise that you should jettison trying to look normal, which makes many of those disabled people compare themselves with so-called normal people.

Disabled or not, women are more prone than men to invest in appearance, to internalise the thin ideal, and feel pressured from the media (McKay et al., 2018), suggesting having a physical disability does not largely affect the tendency for women to internalise the thin ideal. "You're worth it!" trumpet the ads which portray idealistic images and glory the glitter of beauty enhancing products by the beauty industry.

Argyrides et al.'s final analysis of their Greek study revealed several main findings. First, results showed that as age increases, individuals are less satisfied with their appearance, invest less in it and idealise being thin less. These trends seem to be present in individuals with disabilities as well. The findings also showed that individuals with higher levels of inhibition as a result of their disability have low levels of satisfaction with their appearance and low self-esteem.

Finally, results found that appearance satisfaction, self-esteem, and situational body image dysphoria were inversely related to negative perceptions of the disability by others. How others see us matters. This is backed up by previous research in which Taleporos and McCabe (2002) suggest that individuals with physical disabilities tend to internalise the perceptions of others towards their disability, whether negative or positive, affecting their body image satisfaction. This is significant because not only can negative perceptions have a negative effect on body image issues, but positive perceptions and supportive attitudes can promote body image satisfaction and acceptance. These findings highlight the significance of a supportive social environment in supporting individuals with physical disabilities.

11 The Significance of Hair on Body Image

A change of scene. Sigmund Freud has come to the barbers in Vienna. It is called Sweeney Todski. He is accompanied by a rabbi.

BARBER: How do you like your hair cut Dr Freud?
FREUD: Do you have any children?
BARBER: You know I don't.
FREUD: Fathers want to castrate their sons. That is why when I sit in your chair I am accompanied by a rabbi.
BARBER: Have I ever hurt you?
FREUD: There is always a first time. You call your salon Sweeney Todski. Sweeney Todd was a barber who killed all his clients. And baked them in pies.
BARBER: He was English was he not? But he made them pay before he cut their...
FREUD: Throats. You hesitate to say the word.
(Freud bounds out of the chair. He and the rabbi put the barber in the chair.)
RABBI: I often circumcise boys. You do the throat, and I'll do the penis.

This macabre little fantasy is a way of introducing the role of hair in the unconscious.

In his book *The Unconscious Significance of Hair,* Charles Berg examines hair issues very carefully in the light of dreams, anthropology, folklore, symptoms and perversions. He shows them to be an expression of instinct-driven tensions and conflicts.

Berg says that unkept, growing hair symbolises giving in to aggressive libidinal urges. Cutting is a symbol of castration, and conflicts are displaced to hair. And hair often has sexual associations. It reflects conscious, explicit desires. For example, I say I'm shaving my head

DOI: 10.4324/9781003425878-11

because I have decided to become celibate. This is not unconscious desire.

There are interesting Pacific parallels.

For example, a Trobriander, a person who lives in Papua New Guinea shaves his head after his relative dies.

But this is not a spontaneous expression of grief, as Berg argues. His thesis might be put as: "When the mourner shaves his head he is saying symbolically "I loved the deceased." Rather, it is a calculated message to others to say, "I loved the deceased, and I didn't kill him through sorcery."

The famous anthropologist Malinowski wrote: "All those who are suspected of hostile intentions against the deceased are required to make symbolic gesture which says, "I love the deceased."

Head shaving is a public symbol with an explicit message.

The difference is that for Berg it expresses the actual psychological state while for Malinowski it is about what they should feel.

For the psychoanalyst, hair symbolises power because the beholder has an Oedipus complex. For the anthropologist, hair symbolises power because it represents the power of God. So, Berg cannot say that anthropological evidence supports his argument.

Shaving and hair removal

Ancient Egyptians were obsessive about hygiene, and the upper classes often bathed many times each day. They believed that body hair was a sign of uncleanliness, so both men and women removed every trace of it from the body – head to toe! In some cases, caustic ingredients like quicklime and arsenic were used in these primitive depilatory creams and shaving lotions. Early razors also appeared around the time. They would shave their heads completely bald, and then design cooling wigs to wear out in public.

The fear of uncleanliness may have been the early reason for prehistoric man to shave as well. Body hair provides an ideal environment for lice and other unwanted critters and can also be a breeding ground for fungal infections, particularly in hot or humid weather. Egyptians shaved to keep out bugs before Jehovah smote them with lice. Too much hair made you smell which is why the Egyptians used perfume and developed shaving.

Having an unshaven face in Egypt meant that you could not afford to visit a barber every day, or perhaps that you didn't care about your appearance or standing in society.

Shaving wasn't immediately embraced by the rest of the world, but the Greeks and Romans were eventually won over in the 4th century BCE.

Alexander the Great advocated shaving – every single day – but also noted that less hair meant enemy combatants would have less to grab onto, making his soldiers hardier and more formidable.

For the next thousand years, shaving spread throughout Europe, the Middle East, and Asia. Some cultures revelled in a clean but impressive beard, while shaving off all the other hair on their bodies, while other cultures kept their face and head meticulously smooth but did not remove body hair in other areas.

For such a global trend, there have been surprisingly few major advances, although the widespread use of a "hoe-style" razor instead of a straight razor does make the process far easier, so you do not have to sit in the barber's chair. Disposable razors in the late 19th century improved the quality of every shave and eliminated the need for leather strops and honing stones.

Today, the world has changed yet again, and in the past decade we have seen a massive resurgence in growing of long beards. Marx had one but then he came from a family of rabbis. Hair on other parts of the body have had similar periods of rising and falling popularity. The question of shaving between genders remains a controversial and oft-discussed topic.

Women and Shaving

For thousands of years, most women didn't show off their bare arms or their underarms, so those areas remained unshaven. Once it became socially appropriate to show those areas, cultural and aesthetic judgments were made about the presence of hair on the underarms.

Men, however, did not have such a taboo about showing their underarms, nor did they typically shave that part of their body in the past two millennia.

The traditional idea of beauty for women has shifted and there is intense social pressure to conform to that ideal of beauty, whether it is shaving your legs because pantyhose is in style or shaving your pubic area because that's "what men like."

At least in America and parts of Europe, seeing hair under a woman's arms is once again becoming common, while the practice of shaving one's legs is being widely questioned even though advertisers offer women's razors.

Unwanted hair

Excessive or unwanted hair that grows on a woman's body and face is the result of hirsutism. The main difference between typical fine hair on a woman's body and face (often called "peach fuzz") and hair caused by hirsutism is the texture. Excessive hair is usually coarse and dark.

Women with this condition have characteristics that are commonly associated with male hormones, higher-than-normal levels of androgens, including testosterone. All women produce androgens, but the levels typically remain low. Certain medical conditions can cause a woman to produce too many androgens. This can cause them to grow hair like men and to develop other male characteristics, such as a deep voice.

Hirsutism affects between 5 and 10 per cent of women and tends to run in families. Women of Mediterranean, South Asian, and Middle Eastern heritage are also more likely to develop the condition.

Polycystic ovarian syndrome (PCOS) accounts for three out of every four hirsutism cases. Cysts that form on the ovaries can affect hormone production, leading to irregular menstrual cycles and decreased fertility.

The Office of Women's Health DATE states that women with PCOS often have moderate-to-severe acne and tend to be overweight.

Additional symptoms can include fatigue, mood changes, infertility, pelvic pain, headaches, and sleep problems.

Cures for hirsutism can include losing weight if you're overweight – which can help control hormone levels- hair removal creams or bleaching, a prescription cream to slow hair growth on your face and taking a contraceptive pill. There are also treatments that can get rid of unwanted hair for longer than the things you can do at home. However, they are not usually available on the National Health Service and can be expensive. They include laser hair removal and electrolysis – where an electric current is used to stop your hair growing.

Beards

Nigel Barber, using data on British facial hair trends between 1842 and 1971 found that men with beards and moustaches increased as the number of women old enough to marry decreased. Basically, if there are more single men than women, more men grow beards. So, does this mean men grow beards because women find them more attractive than clean-shaven baby faces?

A number of studies suggest that both men and women find that men with beards look older, stronger and more aggressive than non-bearded men. But does that make them more attractive?

Some studies find that women prefer the rough diamond look with stubble (even when kissing), while others show that women like fully bearded men and some even suggest women find clean-shaven men the most attractive. There is no conclusive data suggesting that women find men with facial hair more attractive than clean-shaven men.

The lack of consistent evidence means that we cannot assume men grow beards because women find them more attractive. But if not for women, then why grow a beard?

Across the animal kingdom, the dominant male can get more mating opportunities by intimidating other suitors to step aside. Since men with beards are perceived by both sexes as older, stronger, and more aggressive, the bearded man has an upper hand in perceived dominance, and therefore an increased likelihood of passing his genes on to the next generation. So, from an evolutionary perspective, it appears that beards are a sign of dominance and therefore indirectly a means of procreation.

But what about the moustache?

In researching this book, I stumbled upon a bizarre and irresistible topic of competitions for the best moustache: what will humans not do to spruce up their body image?

I have also found a mug which is decorated with the moustache galaxy. The mug illustrates the 16 traditional categories of judgement in The World Beard and Moustache Championships, arranged in three groups: Moustaches, Partial Beards, and Full Beards. I quote the regulations:

Moustaches

Natural Moustache

Moustache as it grows and left natural. The more natural the better. No closed curls. All hair growing from more than 1.5 cm past the corner of the mouth must be shaved. The moustache may be maintained but without styling aids.

Dali Moustache

Slender with the tips curled upward. Hairs growing from beyond the corner of the mouth must be shaved. The tips may not extend above the level of the eyebrows.

English Moustache

The hairs extend outward from the middle of the upper lip. The tips may be slightly raised. Hairs growing from beyond the corner of the mouth must be shaved.

Imperial Moustache

Small and bushy with the tips curled upward. Hairs growing from beyond the corner of the mouth must be shaved. Styling aids permitted.

Hungarian Moustache

Big and bushy. The hair extends outward from the middle of the upper lip. All hair growing from more than 1.5 cm past the past the corner of the mouth must be shaved. Otherwise, your goulash will trickle into your moustache.

Freestyle Moustache

All moustaches not meeting the criteria for other categories may compete in this category. All hair growing from more than 1.5 cm past the corner of the mouth must be shaved.

Partial Beard

Goatee Natural

The goatee appears as it grows naturally. The more natural the better!

The goatee and moustache may be maintained but without any styling aids. The moustache may not be curled. An area at least 4 cm wide (the width of a razor blade) between the temple and the goatee must be clean shaven.

Musketeer

The beard is narrow and pointed. The moustache is slender, long, and drawn out in a slight bow. The moustache may not include hairs growing from more than 1.5 cm past the corners of the mouth.

Fu Manchu

All areas more than 2cm past the corner of the mouth must be clean shaven, as must all areas under the chin. The tips of the moustache extend downward. The Genghis Khan moustache style is also acceptable.

Goatee Freestyle

Free design and styling of the goatee. All goatees not meeting the criteria for other categories may compete in this category. An area at least 4 cm wide (the width of a razor blade) between the temple and the goatee must be clean shaven.

Imperial Partial Beard/Kaiser Beard

Hair on the cheeks and upper lip. There must be clean shaven spaces of at least 4 cm wide (the width of a razor blade) on the chin and between the facial hair and the onset of the head hair. The whiskers are styled upwards. No closed curls. The hairs on the upper lip may not be separated from the hairs on the cheeks. The hairs may not be too long, not above the level of the eyes.

Partial Beard Freestyle and Sideburns

Free design and styling of all partial beards that are not goatees. Such partial beards not meeting the criteria for other categories may compete in this category. An area at least 4 cm wide (the width of a razor blade) between the temple and the goatee must be clean shaven. Areas at least 4 cm wide (the width of a razor blade) on the chin and between the temple and the goatee must be clean shaven.

The Sideburns category was introduced for the Carson City worlds in 2003 to honour the King, Elvis Presley. The Association of German Beard Clubs translates the name of this category into English as "Whiskers 'Freestyle' & 'Sideburns'," but the German description excludes sideburns – a term not used in German and a facial hair style not common in Germany.

Full Beard Natural

The beard appears as it grows naturally. The more natural the better! The moustache may not be highlighted. The beard may not be curled under at the bottom!

Full Beard Styled Moustache

The moustache is distinct from the beard but may not include hair growing from more than 1.5 cm past the corner of the mouth. The moustache may be styled as in the Dali, English, Hungarian, and Imperial moustache categories.

The beard appears as it grows and left natural. The more natural the better!

Verdi

Full beard, short and rounded at bottom, no more than 10 cm in length as measured from the bottom of the lower lip. The moustache is distinct from the beard but may not include hair growing from more than 1.5 cm past the corner of the mouth.

You have to sing an aria when combing it.

Garibaldi

The beard is wide and rounded at the bottom, and no more than 20 cm in length as measured from the bottom of the lower lip. The beard appears as it grows naturally. The more natural the better. The moustache may not be made distinct from the beard or styled. The beard may not be curled under at the bottom.

Garibaldi is also a biscuit. Try not to get crumbs in your beard when you snack on it.

12 Baldness and Hair Trauma

By the age of 50, half of all men will have noticeable hair loss. By the age of 60 around two thirds will be getting there. Male baldness may be common, but it causes men distress and anguish. It's strongly associated with the development of depression, anxiety, and poor self-image.

Baldness reminds us of our mortality. It speaks on a deep level to how we perceive ourselves and how we think others view us. There is a sense of powerlessness and impotence: single men often worry that they will never find a partner, and those with a partner worry that their partners will stop finding them attractive. And find a hairy replacement.

A multi-billion-pound industry promises a lot but tends not to deliver. I particularly like X FREE FASTGroTM Herbal Hair Treatment, which costs a mere $324. You can use it on your scalp and also in your cooking as it contains premium Chinese herbs like ginseng, dang gui, and he shou wu, to help you "achieve the hair of your dreams with absolutely no downtime or side effects! And why not shampoo what you have left with newt-o-magic?

There is no magic pill or miracle surgery to reverse hair loss. But there are options. The two most common medications are minoxidil (Rogaine) and finasteride (Propecia). Scientists originally developed minoxidil to treat high blood pressure. They found that it had the side effect of excessive, unwanted hair growth. So, drug companies have tried it to cure male baldness.

Researchers do not know exactly how minoxidil works. It appears to widen the hair follicles, which causes thicker strands of hair to grow.

Minoxidil also appears to prolong the growth period of hair. It is approved by the Food and Drug Administration (FDA) only for the treatment of androgenetic alopecia in males and females.

DOI: 10.4324/9781003425878-12

Minoxidil can cause some side effects:

- hair shedding, which seems contradictory
- skin irritation and redness
- itchy, yellow, or white scales on the scalp
- allergic contact dermatitis
- excessive hair growth over the body, including on the face in some women.

And don't expect instant results. It may take 2–4 months for a person to see results.

Finasteride

Finasteride is also an FDA-approved treatment. Scientists originally created it to treat prostate cancer. It works by decreasing the amount of the hormone dihydrotestosterone (DHT) in the scalp. DHT appears to cause hair follicles on the scalp to become thinner, so reducing DHT levels may promote hair regrowth and slow hair loss.

This drug is suitable only for adult males and is not suitable for people who are pregnant or nursing. Possible side effects of finasteride include:

- erectile dysfunction
- decreased libido
- decreased ejaculate volume
- depression

Patience is needed too. Individuals may not experience noticeable results until they have been using the product for three months.

Platelet-Rich Plasma (PRP) injection is a newer treatment that doctors use for androgenetic alopecia. It involves a doctor taking a blood sample and running it through a centrifuge machine. This machine separates the PRP in the blood so the doctor can extract the platelets and inject them into specific areas of a person's scalp. The platelets may promote healing in damaged hair follicles.

According to a 2019 review, PRP therapy can reduce hair loss, but the research supporting this is of low quality. This treatment is not FDA-approved.

The only surgery available to address hair loss is hair transplant surgery, which involves removing hair follicles from the back of the head, where they are resistant to DHT, and placing them on the scalp.

The American Society of Plastic Surgeons warns though that the risks of hair transplant surgery include excessive bleeding and wide scars. Additionally, the skin plugs may die, and this requires further surgery to fix.

Laser treatments, such as combs, are a newer form of hair loss treatment. Advocates claim that these devices promote hair growth by using concentrated light to stimulate hair follicles.

A 2019 study found that a novel laser cap improved hair density and diameter, as well as the visual thickness of hair, in 19 participants. However, the authors note several limitations to this study, such as a small sample size.

Alopecia

Some forms of hair loss however can hit anyone – male or female – at any time. There are three main forms, loss: alopecia areata, the partial loss of hair from the head, alopecia totalis, which is the loss of all head hair; and alopecia universalis, the loss of every hair there had been every been on the head and body.

Alopecia is an autoimmune disorder that arises as a combination of genetic and environmental influences (Madani & Shapiro, 2000). The hair follicles in the growth stage of development are attacked. Why they are attacked is – again – not fully understood, but it appears to be a complex relationship between individual characteristics (e.g., immune system problems, personality, coping styles) and the environment (e.g., a stressful situation).

There is an estimated lifetime risk of alopecia of 1.7 per cent (Kalish & Gilhar, 2003), though the actual figure is unknown because many people with alopecia do not go to a doctor. If the figure is accurate, however, it would indicate that around one million people suffer from alopecia in the UK at some point in their life.

Alopecia is neither life-threatening nor painful, though there can be irritation of the skin, weakness of the fingernails, and physical problems resulting from the loss of eyelashes and eyebrows. Eyelashes and brows are surprisingly effective against the rain, and eyelashes help turn the eyelid outwards. Without eyelashes the lids turn in and irritate the cornea, similar to constantly having grit in the eye.

One woman with alopecia, Natasha Manoura, wrote an article for online publication, *The Cut* on 'The Challenge of Enjoying Sex While Wearing a Wig' in 2018. She writes how she has had to live with the worry of her wig coming off at an inopportune moment, and how she made compromises to favour wig-specific sex moves.

> "It took a long time before I was confident enough to think about flirting, kissing, and getting naked in front of another human being with a bunch of synthetic hair on my head. Even now, I haven't figured out how to lose myself to hot, sweaty, hold-onto-your-seats sex without worrying about whether my hair is going to fly off as a result."

On the subject of her partners' reactions to her baldness, Natasha describes how they have not always been diplomatic:

> "Like A, who loudly proclaimed it was weird when I took my wig off in the morning. Or my last boyfriend, J, who thought it was funny to tell me I looked like one of Roald Dahl's Witches. You know, because I have big feet and no hair.
>
> In all these situations, I've found myself silently agreeing with the reactions. For the most part, I like the way my body looks. I work out, and I work out hard, because if I'm going to be bald, then goddamn it, I'm going to get as close as I can to having a six pack. But the confidence I feel when I look in the mirror has never quite made it up to my head."

She described a number of lovers including one man. She ended up on top, but her hair didn't follow. "The ground did not swallow me up, and the two of us had a great night."

And S, in turn, paved the way for her current partner, F. He asked to see her without her wig, felt her head with his warm, comforting hands, and for the next few hours, made her forget "I hadn't put it back on. When we went back to his place, he asked me if I would keep my hair off, but only if I was okay with it. I wasn't, not entirely, but I also wanted to see how I felt if I did. And I felt good. No, great. It was, in all my 33 years, the first time I had been intimate with a man without my wig on. These days, when the hair comes off at night, it's not by accident."

Psychology and alopecia

As that above account shows alopecia can cause intense emotional suffering, and personal, social and work-related problems. Surveys have shown that around 40 per cent of women with alopecia have had marital problems, and around 63 per cent claimed to have career-related problems (Hunt & McHale, 2004).

Alopecia can also lead to depression, anxiety, and social phobia. This relationship between alopecia and psychosocial consequences can be complicated, in that alopecia can result from a stressful experience, and then itself lead to further distress. Limited research has been carried out in the area. It tends to strike at a critical developmental period when young people are becoming adults with a mean age of onset reported between 25.2 and 36.3 years.

There is evidence that stressful life events have an important role in triggering episodes of alopecia (Garcia-Hernandez et al., 1999). Women who experience high stress are 11 times more likely to experience hair loss than those who do not. (York et al., 1998). Compared with the general population, increased prevalence rates of psychiatric disorders are associated with alopecia (Koo et al., 1994) suggesting that people with alopecia may be at higher risk for development of depression, anxiety disorder, social phobia or paranoid disorder.

Egele and Tauschke (1987) identified a group of alopecia patients with an ongoing feeling of loss, suggesting that for some individuals the process of coping with alopecia may be equated with grief following bereavement.

There are also issues relating to self and identity. The loss of hair, particularly the eyelashes and brows which help to define a person's face, means that a person looks very different. Hair loss may be seen as a failure to conform to the norms of physical appearance within society, a situation which may set people apart in their own estimation and in the estimation of others.

Why me?

Hunt and McHale (2005) collected questionnaires and e-mail interviews with individuals with alopecia, ranging in age from 12 to 93 years.

Women are more likely to want to talk about their alopecia because the disorder can be more difficult for them. Put simply, in our Western culture a bald man is socially acceptable, a bald woman is not.

Many participants desperately wanted to find out why they had alopecia and searched everywhere for a cure. Others had issues about their relationships, with some spouses being very supportive, but in some cases the alopecia was the catalyst to end a relationship.

Some people felt they could not go outside or go to work for fear of being mocked. Women in particular described having problems, perhaps because of the importance of hair to a woman's notion of self and identity. Children and adolescents had problems, not just because they might be bullied at school, but because they are the ones going through the stages of establishing identity. If one's physical appearance changes abruptly at this point, then this can have catastrophic consequences.

These findings are similar to those obtained for other types of fundamental appearance change or physical disfigurement, which often have profound psychosocial effects (e.g., Rumsey & Harcourt, 2005). Visible skin disorders having social anxiety and social avoidance implications simply because they are visible, irrespective of any physical problems associated with the disorder.

Treatments for alopecia

There are medical treatments for alopecia, but unfortunately there is no good evidence that they work in the long-term. This is especially true for the more serious types of alopecia but in many cases the problem resolves itself, and any treatment can take three to six months to be effective. Application of corticosteroids is a common treatment though there may be potentially serious side effects if they are taken for a long time. Diphenylcyclopropenone (DPCP) is also used, with varying results – while there is initially some success, there is a high relapse rate (Aghaei, 2005). Minoxidil is also used.

Dobbins (2003) found no good clinical evidence for the effectiveness of any of the treatments. Some studies show that spontaneous regrowth does occur without treatment, particularly with patchy hair loss (alopecia areata), but the studies that have been carried out do not account for this with suitable controls. Furthermore, the treatments can be lengthy and painful, and cease to be effective when stopped.

Alopecia and physical activity

Hair loss may lead to being targeted for ridicule and bullying. Some are very resilient, but some will struggle, and so mental health management via physical activity may help. One study has examined the link between levels of physical activity and scores on measures of anxiety, depression and stress in Australians who have alopecia.

A total of 83 participants responded to the study through the Australia Alopecia Areata Foundation network and the Foundation's social media sites. The International Physical Activity Questionnaire-Short Form (IPAQ-SF) was used to assess levels of physical activity.

Subjects reported the frequency and duration of: (1) vigorous (examples given included heavy lifting, fast bicycling); (2) moderate (carrying light loads and bicycling at a regular pace); and (3) walking activities, as well as the average time spent sitting on a weekday, including sitting at work, during the last seven days. Total moderate to vigorous physical activity was calculated by combining the activity score of both moderate and vigorous intensity activity for each work and recreational activity domain.

Mental health status of the participants was assessed using the Depression and Anxiety Stress Scale (DASS 21) questionnaire which what it says it measures. Anxiety, and Stress. Almost half the 83 participants, reported having body mass index (BMI) in the normal range. Almost half (49.3 per cent) of the participants reported their self-rated health as fair or good, while the rest reported their health as very good or excellent.

Around half of the participants experienced hair loss affecting more than half the scalp (50 per cent and above). 56 per cent reported hair loss affecting eyebrows, eyelashes and pubic areas. More than half of the participants reported extremely severe anxiety and a slightly lower percentage reported being extremely depressed.

A study in the United States found that individuals with alopecia wanted to find alternative ways of coping such as physical activity as they were unhappy with their current medical treatments. More than half had tried exercise, while others tried yoga and other relaxation techniques (50.4 per cent)

Doctors have not capitalised on the positive outcomes of exercise though a study of 236 psychologists revealed that 83 per cent reported often recommending physical activity 67 per cent often provided advice, and 28 per cent often did physical activity counselling.

We need more studies examining the associations of quality of life, mental health and physical activity in larger samples. Doctors should address the needs of individuals specifically. For example, focus group discussions allow researchers to understand the specific preferences and experiences of patients – and what encourages them to keep exercising.

Hair colour and stress

Hair reacts to shock. I have some family history again. In 1952 my great Uncle Joe and his wife went to the airport to wave off their son as he flew back home after a vacation. In front of their eyes his plane crashed.

There were no survivors. Jo's hair turned white that day. He was a tragic example of shock causing hair loss.

Animal experiments help explain sudden changes in hair colour. Studies on mice show stem cells that control skin and hair colour became damaged after intense stress.

In a chance finding, dark-furred mice turned completely white within weeks. U.S. and Brazilian researchers said this was worth exploring further to develop a drug that prevents hair colour loss from ageing.

Men and women can go grey any time from their mid-30s, with the timing of parental hair colour change giving most of the clues on when.

Although it's mostly down to the natural ageing process and genes, stress can also play a role. But scientists were not clear exactly how stress affected the hairs on our heads. Researchers behind the study, published in Nature, from the Universities of Sao Paulo and Harvard, believed the effects were linked to melanocyte stem cells, which produce melanin and determine hair and skin colour.

And while carrying out experiments on mice, they stumbled across evidence this was the case.

Mousy hair

Experiments in mice have shown some encouraging results. When hair follicles were first generated from stem cells that had been isolated from adult mouse skin, Jay Leno – a former host of US talk show The Tonight Show – joked that scientist "cured baldness ... at least in mice." Sixteen years on, the current host will have the opportunity to mention that scientists have 'cured' baldness in humans, now that Lee et al. (2XXX), writing in *Nature*, have regenerated hair follicles from human stem cells. This achievement places us closer to generating a limitless supply of hair follicles that can be transplanted to the scalps of people who have thinning or no hair.

"We now know for sure that stress is responsible for this specific change to your skin and hair, and how it works," says Prof Ya-Cieh Hsu, research author from Harvard University.

'Damage is permanent'

Pain in mice triggered the release of adrenaline and cortisol, making their hearts beat faster and blood pressure rise, affecting the nervous system and causing acute stress.

This process then sped up the depletion of stem cells that produced melanin in hair follicles.

"I expected stress was bad for the body," said Prof Hsu.

"But the detrimental impact of stress that we discovered was beyond what I imagined.

"After just a few days, all of the pigment-regenerating stem cells were lost.

"Once they're gone, you can't regenerate pigment anymore – the damage is permanent."

In another experiment, the researchers found they could block the changes by giving the mice an anti-hypertensive, which treats high blood pressure. And by comparing the genes of mice in pain with other mice, they could identify the protein involved in causing damage to stem cells from stress. When this protein – cyclin-dependent kinase (CDK) – was suppressed, the treatment also prevented a change in the colour of their fur.

This leaves the door open for scientists to help delay the onset of grey hair by targeting CDK with a drug. "These findings are not a cure or treatment for grey hair," Prof Hsu told the BBC.

"Our discovery, made in mice, is only the beginning of a long journey to finding an intervention for people. It also gives us an idea of how stress might affect many other parts of the body," she said.

Eating your hair

Some people develop a neurotic habit, which only makes things worse. Trichotillomania, also known as hair pulling disorder, is the repetitive pulling out of one's hair. You pull, pick, scrape, or bite their hair, skin, or nails, resulting in damage to the body.

About 1 or 2 in 50 people experience trichotillomania in their lifetime. It usually begins in late childhood/early puberty. In childhood, it occurs about equally in boys and girls but 80–90 per cent of reported adult cases are women. Without treatment, trichotillomania tends to be a chronic condition that may come and go throughout a lifetime.

Trichotillomania is currently classified under "Obsessive-Compulsive and Related Disorders" in the *Diagnostic and Statistical Manual of Mental Disorders*, Fifth Edition. The diagnostic criteria include:

- Recurrent hair pulling, resulting in hair loss
- Repeated attempts to decrease or stop the behaviour
- Clinically significant distress or impairment in social, occupational, or other area of functioning
- Not owing to substance abuse or a medical condition like a dermatological issue
- Not better accounted for by another psychiatric disorder

Many individuals report noticeable sensations before, during, and after pulling. Many emotions, spanning from boredom to anxiety, frustration, and depression can affect hair pulling, as can thoughts, beliefs, and values.

Pulling your hair is embarrassing so people may avoid activities and social situations which may lead them to feel vulnerable to being "discovered" (such as windy weather, going to the beach, swimming, doctor's visits, hair salon appointments, childhood sleepovers, readying for bed in a lighted area, and intimacy).

For some people, trichotillomania is a mild problem, merely a frustration. But for others, the shame results in emotional distress which makes them vulnerable to mood or anxiety disorder. Hair pulling can lead to great tension and strained relationships with family members and friends.

If you eat your hair, it can also lead to gastrointestinal distress or to develop a trichobezoar (hairball in the intestines or stomach), which could lead to gastrointestinal blockage and require surgical removal.

Although trichobezoars are rare, they are a serious risk.

13 Body Image as We Age

And as we get older, our body changes. The great poet Thomas Hardy lamented:

I look into my glass,
And view my wasting skin,
And say, "Would God it came to pass
My heart had shrunk as thin!"
For then, I, undistrest
By hearts grown cold to me,
Could lonely wait my endless rest
With equanimity.
But Time, to make me grieve,
Part steals, lets part abide;
And shakes this fragile frame at eve
With throbbings of noontide.

Father William answered Hardy by standing on his head like a young man. Edward Lear, the virtuoso of limericks, took a comic view of ageing:

"You are old, Father William," the young man said,
"And your hair has become very white;
And yet you incessantly stand on your head –
Do you think, at your age, it is right?"

In her poem 'On Aging' (1993), Maya Angelou notes she is still the same person she was when young though she has less hair and less wind.

But it is not only that the bodily signs of old age – wrinkles, grey hair, deafness, perhaps dribbling one's food as Sartre did, a shuffling

DOI: 10.4324/9781003425878-13

walk, that are off-putting. These body image signs are often wrongly taken to reveal the entire 'inner' being of an old person. The stereotype – the old are commonly presumed to be incompetent and unable to do anything useful or socially valuable. They are often spoken to in the condescending, infantilising tones or 'elderspeak.'

Simone de Beauvoir writes in her magisterial study of the topic, *La Vieillesse* (1970) that old age arouses a visceral aversion, often a 'biological repugnance.' Many try to push it as far away as possible, denying that it will ever happen to them.

In fleeing from our own old age, we also try to distance ourselves from those who are already old: they are 'the Other,' a 'foreign species, and as 'outside humanity.' De Beauvoir argues that this "merges with their consuming boredom, with their bitter and humiliating sense of uselessness, and with their loneliness in the midst of a world that has nothing but indifference for them." Beauvoir argues the old are treated as the Other.

She aims to "shatter" what she calls the "conspiracy of silence" surrounding the old for, she insists, if their voices were heard, we would have to acknowledge that these were "human voices."

De Beauvoir claims most societies prefer not to see "abuses, scandals, and tragedies" but that is perverse as we all know we will grow old. So, what causes this failure to face our future, to see the humanity in all human life?

Beauvoir's answer is that famous existentialist phenomenon: bad faith. She is angered by the bad faith of the not-yet-old with respect to the old.

We are duplicitous. On the one hand, many acknowledge that the old deserve respect but on the other hand, "it is in the adult's interest to treat the aged man as an inferior being and to convince him of his decline."

Edward Said's account of his 1979 encounter with Jean-Paul Sartre exemplifies this revulsion – Said was appalled by Sartre's frailty, dependence, and lack of bodily control:

"Sartre's presence, what there was of it, was strangely passive. He said absolutely nothing for hours on end. At lunch he sat looking disconsolate and remaining totally uncommunicative, egg and mayonnaise streaming down his face. I tried to make conversation with him but got nowhere."

More than half a century has passed since de Beauvoir's *La Vieillesse* was published, and many things have changed. Who years ago, could have imagined some heroics during the COVID-19 pandemic such as Captain Tom's walk for charity and the surprising number of old athletes, 90-year-olds now run the marathon – and yet things have also stayed the same. The 'conspiracy of silence' has been replaced by a proliferation of public discourses about the old, who are now more often euphemistically referred to as 'seniors' or 'the elderly.'

The old are expected to dress and act as people of their age 'should' – but that is happening less. Miriam Margoyles is a good example, but attitudes change slowly. De Beauvoir said the old are still treated with a "contempt not unmixed with disgust" that, as Beauvoir puts it, seeks to cast them "outside humanity." In the West at least, that is changing.

De Beauvoir argued we should be willing to listen to the voices of the old – and to work for conditions in which decline and death are not accompanied by this degradation:

> The material needs for flourishing in old age include far more than a generous personal income. Public resources should be greatly extended from their present levels to meet the needs of those (including some younger people, too) who, for example, are deaf, blind, or less mobile.

From redesigning the built environment to create greater access, to establishing more spaces for social participation, to the generous provision of high-quality personal prosthetics, we must work to furnish many such resources. Providing them should not be seen as an unfair 'burden' on the not-yet-old but, rather, as public goods that they too will enjoy in their later years.

"We must stop cheating," Beauvoir writes. "If we do not know what we are going to be, we cannot know what we are; let us recognise ourselves in this old man, or that old woman." She is surely right that what it is to be a human being is at issue in how we see the old. However, recognising ourselves in our older elders is far from easy to achieve, so deep is our fear of old age and so ingrained society's ageism.

Personal Appendix and my own thoughts on ageing

I promised an account of my own body image issues. First, I am straight, but I did like to wear flamboyant clothes – mainly golden harem trousers which I did very off and on till I was fifty. Second, as I have aged, I accept I will never again look like a dashing young man but my ample hair – thank you, Mr. Trichologist – does give me a touch of dash.

Third while I don't jog I'm proud that I can lie on my back and stick my legs 90 degrees up in the air and touch left foot to right foot 66 times at least. On super fit days I do a hundred. Vanity, vanity, OK, which rhymes with inanity and insanity for that matter.

Fourth, I don't diet, but I eat sensibly, which stops me getting fatter.

Finally, I have never used drugs, except since I gave up being an actor when I was 20 and realised I would never be the next Laurence Olivier.

Some answers are obvious. Keep fit, and keep your mind active. Do not get upset when young people don't see you but see only your frailties.

Accept that there are things you can't do as well as you did when you were younger. But there are compensations. Life experiences give you some perspective.

Each local Age UK has its own unique timetable of clubs and classes – what runs at one Age UK will be different to a neighbouring one.

Examples include:

- Arts & Crafts
- Bridge group
- Coffee morning
- Men in sheds
- Photography club
- Pub lunch
- Quizzes
- Tea dance

A popular song gives some of the best advice – If you can't have what you love, love what you have. You have your body. Care for it – after all, it is only body you have. So, accept and enjoy your body image.

References

Body Image

Aghaei, S. (2005). Topical immunotherapy of severe alopecia areata with diphenylcyclopropenone (DPCP): experience in an Iranian population. *BMC Dermatol*, 26(5), 6. doi:10.1186/1471-5945-5-6.

Alleva, J.M., Tracy, L., Tylka, T., Ashley, M., & Van Diest, K. (2017). The Functionality Appreciation Scale (FAS): Development and psychometric evaluation in U.S. community women and men. *Body Image*, 23, 28–44. doi:10.1016/j.bodyim.2017.07.008.

Ambady, N. & Rosenthal, R. (1993). Half a minute: Predicting teacher evaluations from thin slices of nonverbal behavior and physical attractiveness. *Journal of Personality and Social Psychology*, 64, 431–441.

Argyrides, M., Anastasiades, E., & Alexiou, E (2020). Risk and Protective Factors of Disordered Eating in Adolescents Based on Gender and Body Mass Index. *International Journal of Environmental Research and Public Health*, December 10.

Argyrides, M., Koundourou, C., Angelidou, A., & Anastasiades, E. (2023). Body Image, Media Influences, and Situational Dysphoria in Individuals with Visible Physical Disabilities. *Int J Psychol Res (Medellin)*, 16(1), 78–88. doi:10.21500/20112084.6014.

Aristotle. (1998). *The Metaphysics*. London: Penguin.

Bailey, K.A, Cline, K.L., & Gammage, K.L. (2016). Exploring the complexities of body image experiences in middle age and older adult women within an exercise context: The simultaneous existence of negative and positive body images. *Body Image, 6(17)*, 88–99.

Bailey, K.A. & Gammage, K.L. (2020). Applying action research in a mixed methods positive body image program assessment with older adults and people with physical disability and chronic illness. *Journal of Mixed Methods Research*, 14(2), 248–267. doi:10.1177/1558689819871814.

Barber, N. (2024). *The Human Beast*. Independently published.

Beeton, I. (1863). *The Book of Household Management*. See also *Mrs Beeton's Best Bits* by D. Cohen. London: Psychology News (2000).

Bell, R. (1987). *Holy Anorexia*. Chicago, IL: University of Chicago Press.

Berg, C. (2023). *The Unconscious Significance of Hair*. Routledge: London.

Bhandari, S., Winter, D., Messer, D., & Metcalfe, C. (2011). Family characteristics and long-term effects of childhood sexual abuse. *British Journal of Clinical Psychology*, 50(4), 435–451. doi:10.1111/j.2044-8260.2010.02006.x.

Birbeck, D. & Drummond, M. (2003). Body image and the pre-pubescent child. *Journal of Educational Enquiry*, No. 4, 117–127.

Blumberg, M.L. (1975). Psychodynamics of the young handicapped person. *American Journal of Psychotherapy*, 29(4), 466–476.

Bödicker, C., Reinckens, J., Höfler, M., & Hoyer, J. (2022). Is childhood maltreatment associated with body image disturbances in adulthood? A systematic review and meta-analysis. *Journal of Child & Adolescent Trauma*, 15(3), 523–538. doi:10.1007/s40653-021-00379-5.

Bourdieu, P. (1984). *Distinction: A Social Critique of the Judgment of Taste*. London: Routledge and Kegan Paul.

Brown, T.A., Cash, T.F., & Mikulka, P.J. (1990). Attitudinal body-image assessment: Factor analysis of the Body-Self Relations Questionnaire. *Journal of Personality Assessment*, 55(1–2),135–144. doi:10.1080/00223891.1990.9674053.

Bulik, C. et al. (2008). The Genetics of Anorexia Nervosa Collaborative Study: Methods and Sample Description. *Int J Eat Disord., 41(4)*, 289–300. doi:10.1002/eat.20509.

Carroll, L. (1865). *Alice In Wonderland*. Appleton.

Carter, B.T & Luke, S.G. (2020). Best practices in eye tracking research. *International Journal of Psychophysiology*, 155, 49–62. doi:10.1016/j.ijpsycho.2020.05.010.

Cash, T.C. (2001). *The Body Image Workbook*. New Harbinger Publications.

Christie, A. (2008). *Dumb Witness Harper Collins*. London.

Cohen, D. (1997). *Arthur Kavanagh M.P.* London: Psychology News Press.

Cohen, D. (2004). *Death of a Goddess*. Random House, London.

Colette. (2019). *Cheri*. London: Dover Publications.

Cromer, B., Eurile, B., & McCoy, K. (2008). Knowledge, Attitudes And Behavior Related To Sexuality In Adolescents With Chronic Disability. *Developmental Medicine & Child Neurology*, 32(7), 602–610. doi:10.1111/j.1469-8749.1990.tb08544.x.

Cuzzolaro, M., Vetrone, G., Marano, G., & Garfinkel, P.E. (2005). The Body Uneasiness Test (BUT): development and validation of a new body image assessment scale. *Eat Weight Disord*, 11(1), 1–13. doi:10.1007/BF03327738.

Dearborn, G. (1918). *The Psychology of Clothing*. Reissued by Legare Street Press, 2022.

De Beauvoir, S. (1970). *La Vieillesse*. Paris: Gallimard.

Dobbins (2003). doi:10.1177/105566561876966.

Dolto, F. (2023). *The Unconscious Body Image Routledge*. London.

Donne, J. (2006). "To his Mistress Going to bed" in *Selected Poems*. London: Penguin.

Drummond, M. & Philips, J. (2001). An investigation into the body image perception, body satisfaction and exercise expectations of male fitness leaders: implications for professional practice. *Leisure Studies*, 20, 95–105.

Dyer, A., Borgmann, E., Feldmann, R.Jr, Kleindienst, N., Priebe, K., Bohus M., & Vocks, S. (2013). *Body image disturbance in patients with borderline personality disorder: impact of eating disorders and perceived childhood sexual abuse. Body Image*, 10(2), 220–225. doi:10.1016/j.bodyim.2012.12.007.

Eagles, J., Johnson, M., & Millar, H. (1997). A case-control study of family composition in anorexia nervosa. *International Journal of Eating Disorders*, 38(1), 49–54.

Eccleston, M. (1997). *Pushing the Limits*. London: Psychology News Press.

Egele, U.T. & Tauschke, E. (1987). Alopecia—a psychosomatic disease picture? I. Review of the literature. *Psychother Psychosom Med Psychol*, 37(1), 31–35.

Fardouly, J. & Vartanian, L.R. (2016). Social media and body image concerns: Current research and future directions. *Current Opinion in Psychology*, 9, 1–5. doi:10.1016/j.copsyc.2015.09.005.

Fardouly, J., Diedrichs, P., Vartaniana, L.R, & Halliwell, E. (2015). Social comparisons on social media: The impact of Facebook on young women's body image concerns and mood. *Body Image*, 13, 38–45. doi:10.1016/j.bodyim.2014.12.002.

Farrell, A. (2011). *Fat Shame Stigma and the Fat Body in American Culture. Examining the impact of daily exposure to body-positive and fitspiration Instagram content on young women's mood and body image: An intensive longitudinal study*. New York: New York University Press.

Farrell, C., Shafran, R., & Lee, M. (2006). Empirically Evaluated Treatments for Body Image Disturbance: A Review. *European Eating Disorders Review*, 14(5), 289–300. doi:10.1002/erv.693.

Felitti, V., Anda, R.F., Nordenberg, D., Williamson, D., Spitz, A., Edwards, V., Koss, M, & Marks, J. (1998). Relationship of childhood abuse and household dysfunction to many of the leading causes of death in adults. The Adverse Childhood Experiences (ACE) Study. *Am J Prev Med*, 14(4), 245–258. doi:10.1016/s0749-3797(98)00017-8.

Feusner, J., Moody, T., & Hembacher, B. (2001). Abnormalities of Visual Processing and Frontostriatal Systems in Body Dysmorphic Disorder.

Feusner, J. et al. (2010). Inverted Face Processing in Body Dysmorphic Disorder. *J Psychiatr Res*, 44(15), 1088–1094. doi:10.1016/j.jpsychires.2010.03.015.

Field A.E., CamargoJr, C.A., Taylor, C., Berkey, C., Roberts, S., & Colditz, G. (2001). Peer, parent, and media influences on the development of weight concerns and frequent dieting among preadolescent and adolescent girls and boys. *Pediatrics*, 107(1), 54–60. doi:10.1542/peds.107.1.54.

Fiorvanti, G., Svicher, A., & Casale, S. (2021). Alopecia areata, stress and psychiatric disorders: a review. *J. Dermatology*, *25*(*12*), 625–632. https://doi.org/10.1177/14614448211038904.

García-Hernández, M., Ruiz-Doblado, S., Rodriguez-Pichardo, A., & Camacho, F. (2015). Alopecia Areata, Stress and Psychiatric Disorders: A Review. *The J of Dermatology*, 26, 625–632.

Goffman, E. (1963). *Stigma: Notes on the management of spoiled identity*. Prentice Hall.

Goffman, E. (1990). *Stigma*. London: Penguin.

Goffman, E. (2022). *The Presentation of the Self in Everyday Life*. London: Penguin.

Gouveia, M.J., Frontini, R. Canavarro, M.C., & Moreira, H. (2014). Quality of life and psychological functioning in pediatric obesity: the role of body image dissatisfaction between girls and boys of different ages. *Qual Life Res, 23*(9), 2629–2638. doi:10.1007/s11136-014-0711-y.

Grant, J.E., Kim, S.W., & Crow, S.J. (2001). Prevalence and clinical features of body dysmorphic disorder in adolescent and adult psychiatric inpatients. *Journal of Clinical Psychiatry*, 62, 517–522.

Grant, J.E., Kim, S.W., & Eckert, E. (2002). Body dysmorphic disorder in patients with anorexia nervosa: prevalence, clinical features, and delusionality of body image. *Int J Eat Disord*, 32(3), 291–300. doi:10.1002/eat.10091.

Gramich, K. (2013). Caught in the Triple Net? Welsh, Scottish, and Irish Women Writers. In: Joannou, M. (Ed.) *The History of British Women's Writing, 1920–1945. The History of British Women's Writing*. London: Palgrave Macmillan. doi:10.1057/9781137292179_13.

Graves, R. (2007). *Greek Myths*. London: Penguin.

Grogan, S. (2017). *Body Image*. Routledge.

Grogan, S. & Richards, H. (2002). Body image: Focus groups with boys and men. *Men and Masculinities*, 4(3), 219–232. doi:10.1177/1097184X02004003001.

Guest, E., Costa, B., Williamson, H., Meyrick, J., Halliwell, E., & Harcourt, D. (2019). The effectiveness of interventions aiming to promote positive body image in adults: A systematic review. *Body Image*, 30, 10–25. doi:10.1016/j.bodyim.2019.04.002.

Guest, E., Zucchelli, F., Costa, R.B., Halliwell, E., & Harcourt, D. (2022). A systematic review of interventions aiming to promote positive body image in children and adolescents. *Body Image*, 42,(September), 58–74.

Gull, W. (2019). *Collected Published Writings*. Hansebooks.

Hanna, M. & Strober, L.B. (2020). Anxiety and depression in Multiple Sclerosis (MS): Antecedents, consequences, and differential impact on well-being and quality of life. *Mult. Scler. Relat. Disord*, 44, 102261.

Hartmann, A.S., Thomas, J.J., Wilson, A.C., & Wilhelm, S. (2013). Insight impairment in body image disorders: Delusionality and overvalued ideas in anorexia nervosa versus body dysmorphic disorder. *Psychiatry Res*, 210, 1129–1135.

Heider, N., Spruyt, A., & De Houwer, J. (2015). Implicit beliefs about ideal body image predict body image dissatisfaction. *Front Psychol*, 8(6),1402. doi:10.3389/fpsyg.2015.01402.

Hogan, M.J. & Strasburger, V.C. (2008). Body Image, Eating Disorders, and the Media. *Adolesc Med, 19(2008)*, 521–546.

Holden, A. (1993). *Diana's Revenge*. Vanity Fair.

House of Commons survey (2023). Accessibility of products and services to disabled people Fourth Report of Session 2023–24 Report, together with formal minutes relating to the report Ordered by the House of Commons to be printed March 6, 2024. HC 605. Published on March 19, 2024 by authority of the House of Commons.

Howell, G. (2015). *In Vogue*. Penguin.

Hughes, E.K. & Gullone, E. (2011). Emotion regulation moderates relationships between body image concerns and psychological symptomatology. *Body Image*, 8(3), 224–231.

Hunt, N. & McHale, S. (2004). *Coping with alopecia*. London: Sheldon Press.

Hunt, N. & McHale, S. (2005). Reported experiences of persons with alopecia areata. *Journal of Loss and Trauma*, 10, 33–50.

Hunt, N. & McHale, S. (2005). The psychological impact of alopecia. *BMJ*, 331(7522), 951–953.

Janet, P. (2005). *Obsessions et Psychathenie Les Nevroses*. Paris: PRB.

Jankauskienė, R. & Bacevižienė, M. (2020). The Role of Body Image, Disordered Eating and Lifestyle on the Quality of Life in Lithuanian University Students. *International Journal of Environmental Research and Public Health*, 17(5), 1593. doi:10.3390/ijerph17051593.

Johnson, M. (2022). Is dieting Ruining Your Life? The Savvy Psychologist. *Psychology Today*.

Kalish, R.S. & Gilhar, A. (2003). Alopecia areata: autoimmunity—the evidence is compelling. *J Investig Dermatol Symp Proc*, 8(2),164–167. doi:10.1046/j.1087-0024.2003.00802.x.

Kelly, A., Vimalakanthan, K., & Mille, K.E. (2011). Self-compassion moderates the relationship between body mass index and both eating disorder pathology and body image flexibility. *Body Image*, 11, 446–453.

Kelly, J.A. (1983). *Treating child-abusive families: Intervention based on skills-training principles*. New York: Plenum Press.

Kettl, P., Zarefoss, S., Jacoby, K., Garman, C., Hulse, C., Rowley, F., Corey, R., Sredy, M., Bixler, E., & Tyson, K. (1991). Female sexuality after spinal cord injury. *Sexuality and Disability*, 9(4), 287–295. doi:10.1007/BF01102017.

Kleck, R.E. & DeJong, W. (1983). Physical disability, physical attractiveness, and social outcomes in children's small groups. *Rehabilitation Psychology*, 28(2), 79–91. doi:10.1037/h0090997.

Kobo, A. (1964). *The Face of Another*. Tokyo: Kodansha.

Kostanski, M. & Gullone, E. (1995). Adolescent body image dissatisfaction: relationships with self-esteem, anxiety, and depression controlling for body mass. *J of Clinical Child Psych*, 39, 255–262.

Lamarche, L., Bailey, K., Awan, A., Risdon, C., Pauw, G., & Vinoski, T.E. (2020). Exploring primary care providers' understandings of body image in patient care. *Body Image*, 35, 161–170. doi:10.1016/j.bodyim.2020.09.001.

Lambrou, C., Veale, D., & Wilson, G. (2006). Appearance concerns comparisons among persons with body dysmorphic disorder and nonclinical controls with and without aesthetic training. *Journal of Abnormal Psychology*, 120, 443–453.

Larsen, S.E., Fleming, C.J.E., & Resick, P.A. (2019). Residual symptoms following empirically supported treatment for PTSD. *Psychological Trauma: Theory, Research, Practice and Policy*, 11(2), 207–215. doi:10.1037/tra0000384.

Lawrence, C. & Thelen, M. (1991). Body image, dieting, and self-concept: Their relation in African-American and Caucasian children.

Lee, J., Rabbani, C. C., Gao, H., Steinhart, M. R., Woodruff, B. M., Pflum, Z. E., Kim, A. Heller, S., Liu, Y., Shipchandler, T. Z., & Koehler, K. R. (2020). Hair-bearing human skin generated entirely from pluripotent stem cells. *Nature, 582*(7812), 399–404.

Levine, M.P. & Harrison, K. (2004). Media's Role in the Perpetuation and Prevention of Negative Body Image and Disordered Eating. In J.K. Thompson (Ed.), *Handbook of eating disorders and obesity* (pp. 695–717). John Wiley & Sons.

McKay, A., Moore, S., & Kubik, W. (2018). Western beauty pressures and their impact on young university women. *International Journal of Gender and Women's Studies*, 6(2), 1–11.

Mackelprang, R.W. (1993). A holistic social work approach to providing sexuality education and counselling for persons with severe disabilities. *Journal of Social Work & Human Sexuality*, 8(2), 63–87. doi:10.1300/J291v08n02_04.

Mair, C. (2018). *The Psychology of Fashion*. London: Routledge.

Maroto Expósito, P., Hernández López, M., & Valverde, M. (2015). Assessment of Implicit Anti-Fat and Pro-Slim Attitudes in Young Women Using the Implicit Relational Assessment Procedure. *International Journal of Psychology and Psychological Therapy*, 15(1), 17–32.

Marwick, A. (1989). *Beauty in history*. London: Thames & Hudson.

Mendo S., del Rio, M., Amado, D. & Iglesias, D. (2017). Self-Concept in Childhood: The Role of Body Image and Sport Practice. *Frontiers in Psychology*, 8, 853. doi:10.3389/fpsyg.2017.00853.

Michopoulos, V., Powers, A., Moore, C., Villarreal, S., Ressler, K.J., & Bradley, B. (2015). The mediating role of emotion dysregulation and depression on the relationship between childhood trauma exposure and emotional eating. *Appetite*, 91, 129–136. doi:10.1016/j.appet.2015.03.036.

Mikes, G. (1946). *How to be an Alien*. London: Andre Deutsch.

Molloy, D. (2019). Body and Genital Piercing Salamander site. Believe it or not.

Morton, R. (1698). *A Treatise on Consumption*. London: Printed for Richard Wellington ... Arthur Bettesworth ... and Bernard Lintott.

Murphy J.A. & Perez, F. (2002). A Postmodern Analysis of Disabilities. *Journal of Social Work in Disability & Rehabilitation*, 1(3). doi:10.1136/bmj.331.7522.951.

Murray, S. (2023). *Medical Humanities and Disability Studies In/Disciplines Bloomsbury Academic*. London.

Naqvi, I. & Kamal, A. (2017). Translation and validation of multidimensional body self-relation questionnaire-appearance scale for young adults. *Pakistani J of Psychological research*, (December).

Nelson, M. & Gruver, G.G. (1978). Self-esteem and body-image concept in paraplegics. *Rehabilitation Counselling Bulletin*, 22(2), 108–113.

Netemeyer, R.G., Burton, S., & Lichtenstein, D.R. (1995). Trait aspects of vanity: Measurement and relevance to consumer behavior. *Journal of Consumer Research*, 21, 612–626.

Orbach, S. (2016). *Fat is a Feminist Issue*. London: Arrow.

O'Toole, A., LoParo, D., & Craihead x (2021). *A Self-compassion and dissonance-based interventions for body image distress in young adult women Body Image*, 38, 191–200.

Ovid. (2007). *Metamorphoses*. London: Penguin.

Pfaffenberger, N., Gutweniger, S., Kopp, M., Seeber, B., Stürz, K., Berger, T., & Günther, V. (2011). Impaired body image in patients with multiple sclerosis. *Acta Neurol Scand*, 124, 165–170.

Piaget, J. (2001). *The Language and Thought of the Child*. London: Routledge Classics.

Poe, E.A. (2009). *The Murders in the Rue Morgue*. Vintage Classics.

Presnell, K., Bearman, S., & Stice, E. (2004). Risk Factors for Body Dissatisfaction in Adolescent Boys and Girls: A Prospective Study. *International Journal of Eating Disorders*, 36, 389–401. doi:10.1002/eat.20045.

Price, C. (2005). Body-oriented therapy in recovery from child sexual abuse: an efficacy study. *Altern Ther Health Med*, 11(5), 46–57.

Puhl, R. (2022). Weight stigma, policy initiatives, and harnessing social media to elevate activism. *Body Image*, 40, 131–137. doi:10.1016/j.bodyim.2021.12.008.

Puhl, R.M. & Latner, J.D. (2007). Stigma, obesity, and the health of the nation's children. *Psychol Bull*, 133(4), 557–580.

Ravaldi, C. et al. (2003). Eating disorders and body image disturbances among ballet dancers, gymnasium users and body builders. *Psychopathology*, 36(5), 247–254. doi:10.1159/000073450.

Reas, D.L., Whisenhunt, B.L., Netemeyer, R., & Williamson, D.A. (2002). Development of the body checking questionnaire: a self-report measure of body checking behaviors. *Int J Eat Disord*, 31(3), 324–333. doi:10.1002/eat.10012.

Ribiero, B.T. (1964). *Self esteem Coherence in Psychotic Discourse*. Oxford: Oxford University Press.

Ricciardelli, L.A. & McCabe, M.P. (2001). Children's body image concerns and eating disturbance: A review of the literature. *Clinical Psychology Review*, 21(3), 325–344. doi:10.1016/S0272-7358(99)00051–00053.

Rosen, J.C., Srebnik, D., Saltzberg, E., & Wendt, S. (1991). Development of a body image avoidance questionnaire. *Psychological Assessment: A Journal of Consulting and Clinical Psychology*, 3(1), 32–37. doi:10.1037/1040-3590.3.1.32.

Rousso, H. (1992). *Don't Call Me Inspirational*. Temple University Press.

Rumsey, N. & Harcourt, D. (2005). Body image and disfigurement: issues and interventions. doi:10.1016/S1740-1445(03)00005-6.

Scheffers, M., van Busschbach, J.T., Bosscher, R.J., Aerts, L.C., Wiersma, D., & Schoevers, R.A. (2017). Body image in patients with mental disorders: Characteristics, associations with diagnosis and treatment outcome. *Comprehensive Psychiatry*, 74, 53–60. doi:10.1016/j.comppsych.2017.01.004.

Scheffers, M., van Duijn, M.A.J., Bosscher, R., Wiersma, D., Schoevers, R.A., & van Busschbach, J. (2017). Psychometric properties of the Dresden Body Image Questionnaire: A multiple-group confirmatory factor analysis across sex and age in a Dutch non-clinical sample. *PLOS*, July 26. doi:10.1371/journal.pone.0181908.

Schilder, P. (1935). *The Image and Appearance of the Human Body*. Psyche Monographs, no. 4.

Signorelli, N. (1997). Reflections of Girls in the Media: A Content Analysis. A Study of Television Shows and Commercials, Movies, Music Videos, and Teen Magazine Articles and Ads. An Executive Summary. Institute of Education Sciences research paper.

Simmel, G. (1904). *Fashion now in American Journal of Sociology*, 62(6), 541–558. University of Chicago Press.

Skemp, K., Rees, K.S., Mikat, R. & Seebach, E.E. (2006). Body Image Dissatisfaction Among Third, Fourth, and Fifth Grade Children. *Californian Journal of Health Promotion*, 4(3). doi:10.32398/cjhp.v4i3.1958.

Smolak, L. (2004). Body image in children and adolescents: where do we go from here? *Int J Eat Disord*, 36(4), 389–401. doi:10.1002/eat.20045.

Stock, N. & Feragen, K. (2018). Assessing Psychological Adjustment to Congenital Craniofacial Anomalies: An Illustration of Methodological Challenges. *The Cleft Palate Craniofacial Journal*. doi:10.1177/105566561876966.

Stubbs, P. (1597). The Anatomie of Abuses. Internet archive.

Swiatokowki, P. (2016). Magazine influence on body dissatisfaction: Fashion vs. health?. *Cogent Social Sciences*, 2(1). doi:10.1080/23311886.2016.1250702.

Taleporos, G. & McCabe, M.P. (2002). Body image and physical disability—personal perspectives. *Social Science & Medicine*, 54(2002), 971–980.

Thurman, J. (2000). *The Secrets of the Flesh*. London: Bloomsbury.

Tice, L., Hall, R.C., Beresford, T.P., Quinones, J. & Hall, A.K. (1989). Sexual abuse in patients with eating disorders. *Psychiatr Med, 7(4)*, 257–267.

Tiggerman, M. (2004). Body image across the adult life span: stability and change. *Body Image*, 1(1), 29–41. doi:10.1016/S1740-1445(03)00002-0.

UK Disability Survey research report. (2021). An analysis of responses to the UK Disability Survey 2021, and data tables with responses to all questions. Disability Unit.

Vartanian L.R. & Porter A.M. (2016). Weight Stigma and Eating Behavior: A Review of the Literature. *Appetite*, 102ff. doi:10.1016/j.appet.2016.01.034.

Wolman, C., Resnick, M.D., Harris, L.J., & Blum, R.W. (1994). Emotional well-being among adolescents with and without chronic conditions.

Journal of Adolescent Health, 15(3), 199–204. doi:10.1016/1054-139X(94) 90504–90505.
Women's Equality Committee (2021).

Children and young people's mental health

This is a House of Commons Committee report, with recommendations to government. The Government has two months to respond. Eighth Report of Session 2021–22.

Gramich, K. (2018). *The Works of Gwerful Mechain: A Broadview Anthology of British Literature Edition*. Broadview Anthology of British Literature Editions.

Robertson, M., Duffy, F., Newman, E., Prieto Bravo, C., Ates, H.H., & Sharpe, H. (2021). Exploring changes in body image, eating and exercise during the COVID-19 lockdown: A UK survey. *Appetite, 1(159)*, 105062. doi: 10.1016/j.appet.2020.105062.

Samonds, R.J. & Cammermeyer, M. (1989). Perceptions of body image in subjects with multiple sclerosis: a pilot study. *J Neurosci Nurs*, 21(3*), 190–194*.

Children and young people's mental health

This is a House of Commons Committee report, with recommendations to government. The Government has two months to respond. Eighth Report of Session 2021–22. Author: Health and Social Care Committee Date Published: December 9, 2021 by UK Parliament.

INDEX

The perfect index sounds like the title of a story of Borges might have written. I do not claim perfection for this index but it should enable the reader to track down most sources.

For Product Safety Concerns and Information please contact our EU representative GPSR@taylorandfrancis.com
Taylor & Francis Verlag GmbH, Kaufingerstraße 24, 80331 München, Germany

www.ingramcontent.com/pod-product-compliance
Lightning Source LLC
Chambersburg PA
CBHW050523280326
41932CB00014B/2437
* 9 7 8 1 0 3 2 5 4 6 2 8 5 *